MW00623760

SLEEP THROUGH
INSOMNIA

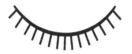 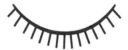

END THE ANXIETY AND
DISCOVER SLEEP RELIEF WITH
GUIDED CBT-I THERAPY

From Verywell's Expert on Sleep

BRANDON R. PETERS, MD

Board-certified in Neurology and Sleep Medicine

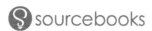

Published by Sourcebooks
P.O. Box 4410, Naperville, Illinois 60567-4410
(630) 961-3900
sourcebooks.com

Originally self-published as *Insomnia Solved* in 2018.

Printed and bound in the United States of America.
POD 10 9 8 7 6 5 4 3 2 1

NOTICE

This publication is designed to provide accurate and authoritative information in regard to the subject matter covered. Care has been taken to confirm the accuracy of the information presented, including that related to current recommendations for drug therapy, and to describe generally accepted practices. It is published with the understanding that the author is not providing medical care to the reader. You should always consult with your physician about any medical conditions. This book and any associated online content and features included (collectively, the "program") do not constitute, and are not a substitute for, medical evaluation, advice, diagnosis, care, or treatment. Brandon Peters, MD, LLC, the provider of the program, recommends that you always seek the advice of a physician or other health care professional for all health-related matters. The program should be used as an educational tool that supports your care and treatment as rendered by your physician. Brandon Peters, MD, as well as Brandon Peters, MD, LLC and its owners, officers, directors, employees, consultants, agents, affiliates, business partners, and licensors will not be liable for, and you waive any claim for, any personal injury, damage, and/or liability arising out of your use of or reliance on the program. Usage of the program is further subject to the Terms of Use Agreement that is accessible to authorized users online at BrandonPetersMD.com.

This book is dedicated to all of the dreamers in this world, to those I have believed in, and to those who have believed in me.

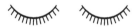

"All men dream: but not equally. Those who dream by night in the dusty recesses of their minds wake up in the day to find it was vanity, but the dreamers of the day are dangerous men, for they may act their dreams with open eyes, to make it possible."

—**T. E. LAWRENCE**,
Seven Pillars of Wisdom: A Triumph

"O sleep! O gentle sleep!
Nature's soft nurse, how have I frighted thee,
That thou no more wilt weigh my eyelids down
And steep my senses in forgetfulness?"

—**WILLIAM SHAKESPEARE**,
Henry IV, Part 2 (act 3, scene i)

Contents

Foreword

Chronic insomnia can devolve into a state of profound desperation. Changes you make may begin to work against you. Fortunately, insomnia is a problem that can be solved. This self-directed program is designed to give you the tools that you need to return your sleep—and life—to normalcy.

Helping someone who has seemingly lost the natural ability to sleep is one of the most satisfying things I do in my profession. Over the short course of 6 weeks, time and time again, I see how cognitive behavioral therapy for insomnia (CBT-I) transforms lives by improving and resolving difficulty sleeping. Patients with decades of insomnia, starting on five different sleeping pills, discover normal sleep without medications in a few short months. "This is a miracle!" they exclaim. "You have made more difference in my life than any doctor I have ever seen," they suggest. "My family says that I am a different person," they observe. Often they wistfully remark, "I wish I had known about this years ago."

There is a growing body of scientific literature that supports the beneficial effects of CBT-I. Sleeping pills have well-known side effects and often lose their efficacy over time. These drugs are associated with confusion, falls, memory problems, and overdose. Due to the potential risks, many physician groups now advocate CBT-I as a more effective alternative.

Unfortunately, there are only a few hundred CBT-I specialists in the United States, many of whom are trained psychologists. Medical doctors, even board-certified sleep medicine physicians, who are trained in CBT-I are extraordinarily rare.

Stanford University trains more board-certified sleep medicine physicians than any other center in the world, but only one per year is formally trained to do CBT-I—only *one*. There are more than 40 million Americans with chronic insomnia. This shortage of CBT-I providers compromises access to the best available treatment, and the disparity is greatest among those who need the help the most. The creation of this resource is born of this great and growing need.

Starting on this path takes a leap of faith. Many people with chronic insomnia feel they have heard, read, and done it all. Nevertheless, their difficulty initiating and maintaining sleep persists. If you had found the right answer, you wouldn't be here. The strong foundation of this program, developed over years based on sound science and professional experience, has helped hundreds of my patients. Trust that it can work for you.

The information provided here must be comprehensive to address diverse needs, yet what may be helpful to you may be very specific and focused. Once discovered, it may seem like common sense, a solution that was elusive becomes second nature. Try to be thorough and attentive in your use of the program, but acknowledge your individual learning style. The content is organized into six weekly lessons around three essential activities:

- Reflection
- Education
- Setting Goals

Each week you will look back at what you have accomplished, build your skill set with additional education, and reinforce the changes you are making through specific planning that ultimately moves you closer to your long-term goals. Do your best to stick to a fixed 6-week schedule.

Everything needed to be successful in this self-directed CBT-I program is included within this book. Not everyone learns best by reading or writing; you may prefer listening to the content, for example. For those who would benefit from additional resources, access is also available to exclusive online content that is integrated into the reading. This content includes a full collection of audio and video files, presentations, and helpful documents. Look for these resources whenever you see the following symbol within the text:

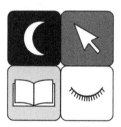

In order to view the secured premium content, it is necessary to register for the full program. Simply go to the online portal and register at: InsomniaSolved.com.

Part of the cost of this book is discounted from the total cost of the program. Simply use the discount code: **PremiumSleep**.

Once registered, click **Log In** and input the time-sensitive password provided via email.

For those who may require additional assistance beyond the scope of this book and the online content, consider one-on-one telemedicine visits to give you a more personalized approach to the program. These resources are likewise available online through the site. You have committed yourself to ending the destructive influence of insomnia; don't hesitate to use the tools needed to once and for all put this problem to bed.

Let the journey to better sleep and health begin.

Dr. Peters

Program Goals and Sleep Needs

Reflection: Health Screening
Education: Normal Sleep, Sleep Needs, and Insomnia
Goal Setting: Program Goals

Learning Objectives:

- Complete a health-related screening questionnaire to identify coexisting sleep, medical, and psychiatric disorders that may interfere with program success.
- Understand the basics of normal sleep, what insomnia is, and the most common causes of insomnia.
- Learn how to use a sleep log to track sleep patterns over the course of the program.

- Establish the ultimate goals to meet upon successful completion of the program.

Health Screening and Exclusions

"Know thyself."
—Temple of Apollo at Delphi

When new patients are first evaluated in my clinic, they complete a comprehensive 4-page intake questionnaire that includes a complete medical history and more than 50 specific queries on sleep. This self-directed program cannot substitute for the skill of a physician who knows you well, someone who can support your efforts and provide guidance. You should always consult with your physician about your medical conditions. You may need to coordinate your participation in this program with their support and advice, especially if you intend to make any changes in your use of sleeping pills.

There are limitations to any intervention and not everyone may be a candidate for participation in a cognitive behavioral therapy for insomnia (CBT-I) program. After years of experience, it is clear that when left untreated, certain medical conditions are associated with higher failure rates. Ignoring a coexisting problem will not make it go away. Instead, striving to complete CBT-I while ignoring a contributing cause is like running a race with a broken leg. There are a variety of medical conditions that should be optimally managed to succeed at CBT-I. Some of these conditions include:

- Anxiety
- Depression
- Bipolar disorder
- Chronic untreated pain
- Fibromyalgia
- Hypothyroidism
- Chronic fatigue syndrome
- Obstructive sleep apnea
- Restless legs syndrome
- Drug or alcohol abuse or withdrawal

Insomnia may be associated with many of these conditions. Just because you have been diagnosed with one of these problems does not mean that you cannot participate in the program. Carefully reflect on what contribution it may have in your situation. If you struggle, revisit its influence on your efforts.

Many people with insomnia question whether it is the right time for them to participate in a CBT-I program. Insomnia often develops in periods of stress. Reflect on whether you are experiencing an acute stress that is likely to resolve in the near future. For example, if you have insomnia while preparing for an examination, and this test is about to occur, it might not be the best time to work at improving your sleep over 6 weeks. You may also wish to defer involvement if you are experiencing a profound recent hardship or stress: divorce, bereavement, job loss, life-changing diagnosis, or personal tragedy. In an extreme analogy, if your house is on fire, don't focus on your sleep. However, if you are experiencing stressors as part of your routine life, and these are unlikely to change in the next few months, now is as good a time as any to get started.

Sleep History

In order to better understand the nature of your sleep problem, take a few minutes to explore some of the prominent features by answering the following questions. These reflections may help to guide you through the program, but they may also serve as a conversation starter with your physician and might prompt further sleep evaluation and testing. Let's start by considering your sleep patterns, with some commentary on why these questions are relevant:

How long have you had your sleep problem?

☐ <1 month   ☐ 1-3 months   ☐ 3-6 months

☐ 6-11 months   ☐ _____ year(s)

_____

_____

_____

Chronic insomnia that responds well to CBT-I occurs at least 3 nights per week and lasts for at least 3 months.

What time do you go to bed?

_____

_____

_____

If you go to bed too early, you may find it is harder to fall asleep, stay asleep, or get back to sleep after waking in the night.

How long does it take you to fall asleep?

_____

It is normal to fall asleep in less than 15 to 20 minutes after turning out the lights.

What do you do if you cannot fall asleep?

When you have difficulty initiating sleep, how you react and what you choose to do can make a difference in whether the insomnia persists.

How many times on average do you wake up in the night?

It is normal to wake up at night, but frequent awakenings can fragment sleep continuity and prolonged time awake at night may undermine sleep quality.

How much time is spent awake?

It is normal to spend less than 30 minutes awake in the night after falling asleep.

What time do you get out of bed in the morning?

Lingering in bed after waking may lead to lighter, fragmented sleep towards morning.

On average, how many hours of sleep do you need to feel rested?

_____

_____

_____

Sleep needs vary based on age, but most adults need 7 to 9 hours of sleep on average each night. Older adults may only need 7 to 8 hours.

On average, how much time are you spending in bed overnight?

_____

_____

_____

If your time in bed exceeds your sleep need, you will spend the difference awake. Too much time in bed, going to bed too early or staying in bed too late, is a common reason that insomnia persists.

What is your preferred sleep timing?

☐ Night Owl   ☐ Morning Lark   ☐ Neither

_____

_____

_____

Night owls commonly have trouble falling asleep and difficulty waking in the morning.

Beyond a better understanding of your sleep patterns, it is also important to recognize signs of other sleep disorders like obstructive sleep apnea and restless legs syndrome that may contribute to insomnia. These conditions may cause awakenings, make it hard to fall asleep or get back to sleep, and lead to other symptoms. Consider some of these questions that may suggest the presence of sleep apnea:

	No	Yes
Do you snore?	☐	☐
Has someone witnessed you stop breathing when you sleep?	☐	☐
Do you wake up gasping or choking or with shortness of breath?	☐	☐
Do you have a dry mouth when sleeping?	☐	☐
Do you grind or clench your teeth at night?	☐	☐
Do you have night sweats?	☐	☐
Do you have heartburn or reflux at night?	☐	☐
Do you get up during the night more than once to urinate?	☐	☐
Do you wake up with palpitations or chest pain?	☐	☐
Do you wake up with a headache in the morning?	☐	☐
Do you have excessive daytime sleepiness or take frequent naps?	☐	☐

The more of the above questions that you answered "Yes" to, the more likely that you may need to consider testing to evaluate for sleep apnea as a contribution to your insomnia. Insomnia secondary to sleep apnea will often manifest as frequent awakenings—especially towards morning—and unrefreshing sleep.

Restless legs syndrome (RLS) may make it hard to fall asleep when first lying down at night. Most people with RLS experience uncomfortable feelings in their legs associated with an urge to move that occurs when lying down at night and is improved by movement. It may also recur after waking in the night. It may require iron replacement or prescription medications to resolve.

If you struggle to adhere to any of the recommendations made as part of this program, especially if daytime sleepiness becomes an impairment, reconsider the role an underlying problem like sleep apnea may play in impeding your progress. Treatment of the coexisting disorder may lead to full resolution of your insomnia. These issues are discussed further in Chapter 5.

Basics of Sleep

Everyone knows what sleep is, but its true nature and role in health continues to be better understood with advances in research. Sleep is defined as a transient and reversible loss of consciousness characterized by decreased responsiveness to the environment. It is required to sustain life. It may have a role in energy conservation, tissue repair, metabolism, memory processing, and optimal daytime function. When sleep quality and quantity are compromised, problems with alertness, concentration, memory, mood, immune function, and metabolism may develop.

An individual's sleep is often assessed with a sleep study called a polysomnogram. This test includes measurement of the electrical activity of the brain. Electrodes are placed on the scalp to measure these patterns with an EEG. Specific stages of sleep can be identified (see Figure 1):

* *Wakefulness* is characterized by high frequency, low amplitude (height) waves as well as body movements, eye blinks, and muscle artifact.

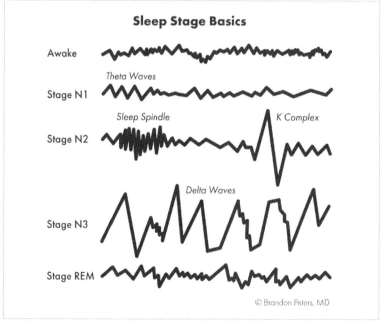

Figure 1

- The lightest state of sleep, called *stage 1 (N1)*, demonstrates a loss of muscle activity and a slowing in the brainwaves called theta activity. Theta is the speed of the waves and these occur at a rate of 5 to 8 times per second (noted in Hertz or Hz). It is during this lightest stage of sleep that unconsciousness begins. However, it is a delicate state, light and unrefreshing, and as many as 50 percent of people will misinterpret stage 1 sleep as wakefulness when awakened.

> As many as 50 percent of people will misinterpret stage 1 sleep as wakefulness.

- *Stage 2 (N2)* is the most common state of sleep and is characterized by findings called sleep spindles and K complexes. These electrical patterns are generated deep within the brain in the thalamus. The brain's surface becomes coordinated, making it harder to wake.

- *Stage 3 (N3) (and previously stage 4)* is the deepest state of sleep, characterized by high amplitude, slow-wave activity. This is also known as delta sleep, named for the waves that occur at 1 to 4 Hz.

- The other major category of sleep is called *Rapid Eye Movement (REM) sleep*. The mind is very active and the electrical activity of the brain appears like wakefulness. The difference is that the body is paralyzed so that dream enactment cannot occur.

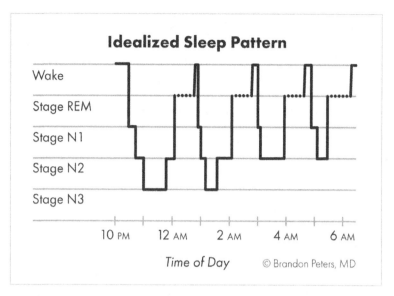

Figure 2

These stages of sleep can be divided into Non-REM and REM sleep. The former accounts for about 75 to 80 percent of the night's sleep for a healthy young adult. REM sleep makes up the remaining 20 to 25 percent. REM sleep tends to occur in cycles every 80 to 110 minutes during the night. It becomes more prolonged towards morning. It is common to wake for the day and interrupt the last period of REM, leading to recall of a vivid dream upon awakening. Sleep evolves in a characteristic pattern (documented with a hypnogram, see Figure 2) with slow-wave sleep predominating in the first 1/3 of the night and REM sleep making up most of the last 1/3. Even though dreams may not be recalled, REM sleep still occurs.

Sleep Changes with Aging

Sleep is a dynamic process, evolving throughout our entire lifespan. Children, adolescents, adults, and the elderly all have dramatically different experiences of sleep. There are distinct sleep needs, proportions of sleep stages, and even sleep quality. To better understand your sleep, it may be helpful to recognize and accept these key differences that are part of normal sleep variation.

Though it is common to say after a good night of sleep that someone "slept like a baby," babies do not actually sleep in a way that would satisfy most adults. Ask any parent who must match a newborn's schedule! A 1-week-old infant may spend more than 16 hours in a 24-hour period asleep, but this sleep is broken up: recurring in short spurts scattered throughout the day and night. This is hard on parents, but usually improves by 3 or 4 months when wakefulness is largely consolidated to the daytime and it becomes possible for the child to sleep better through the night.

Children rarely experience insomnia, and if they do, it may be due to several factors. Some individuals may be predisposed to insomnia from birth with a genetic tendency, and this "primary insomnia" may start to become apparent as a child and persist throughout life. Fortunately, sleep can still be optimized among these individuals with insomnia therapy. Children are also subject to unique behavioral variants of insomnia. Sleep-onset association insomnia occurs in babies who have become conditioned to be held while falling asleep or soothed when waking at night. Toddlers (and even older children) may also have limit-setting insomnia due to resistance in going to bed when the enforcement of a bedtime routine by parents is inadequate. Fortunately, simple interventions—including the Ferber method of graduated extinction—can often improve the sleep of young children. These issues are discussed further within other resources and are beyond the scope of this program.

Sleep changes throughout early childhood and into adolescence (see Figure 3). By the age of 3 years, the average sleep need decreases to 12 hours, with some of it still occurring as daytime napping. By age 4 or 5, the nap goes away, and the amount of sleep needed to feel rested continues to decline through adolescence until it approaches the adult average by age 18. This is only an average, however, and some adults may need more sleep while others can get by on less.

There is variability from one night to the next, and clear changes occur in sleep as we get older (see Figure 4). Stages 1 and 2 are pretty stable as we age, but slow-wave (stage 3) sleep decreases markedly in late adolescence. Growth hormone is released in slow-wave sleep, and once we have reached our adult

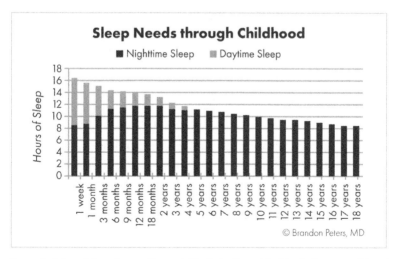

Figure 3: Adapted from Durmer JS, et al. "Pediatric Sleep Medicine." *Continuum. Neurol* 2007;13(3):153–200.

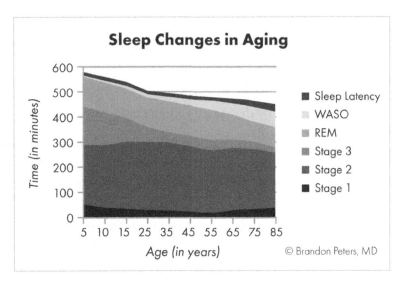

Figure 4: Adapted from Ohayon M, Carskadon MA, Guilleminault C, et al. "Meta-analysis of quantitative sleep parameters from childhood to old age in healthy individuals: developing normative sleep values across the human lifespan." *Sleep* 2004;27:1255–1273.

stature, the stage seems to decrease along with our total sleep needs. As a proportion of our total sleep, REM sleep remains relatively stable throughout life, but may decrease slightly in late life.

There are certain measurements of insomnia that may increase as we become older. **Sleep latency**, the time it takes to fall asleep at the beginning of the night, is stable except in the case of insomnia. It is normal to fall asleep in less than 20 to 30 minutes at the beginning of the night. The amount of time we spend awake at night (known as **wakefulness after sleep onset** or WASO) increases starting in our 30s and even further into our 50s and beyond.

It is normal across a population to spend more time awake at night as we become older. This may occur secondary to other medical conditions that cause chronic pain or due to sleep disorders such as sleep apnea and restless legs syndrome that occur more among older people. Increased insomnia may also be due to a declining ability to sleep or a diminished sleep need. Fortunately, changes can occur to counteract this tendency, such as treating coexisting disorders and reducing time in bed to better match sleep needs.

How Much Sleep Do You Need?

The optimal amount of sleep needed to feel rested varies by individual and can also change as we get older. Most people need 7 to 9 hours of sleep to feel rested, but this is the average for a population (see Figure 5). Some people get by on less sleep and others need more. Determining your sleep needs can help to relieve insomnia.

Research suggests that the average amount of sleep needed to avoid the effects of sleep deprivation is 8 hours and 10 minutes. An "average" person could sleep this much each night and not experience insomnia, desire naps, or have compromised daytime function. This is a bell-shaped curve, however. Just like weight, height, intelligence, and other population-based factors, though there might be an average, there are people at the extremes. You are unlikely to be precisely at this average.

Some people only need 6 hours of sleep (perhaps 2 percent of the population), but just as many may need 10 hours of sleep. The vast majority of the distribution, perhaps 90 percent of people, need 7 to 9 hours of sleep to feel rested. If you are a person with a 10-hour sleep need, you will be sleep deprived if you only get 8 hours of rest. Conversely, if you spend 9 hours in bed but only have

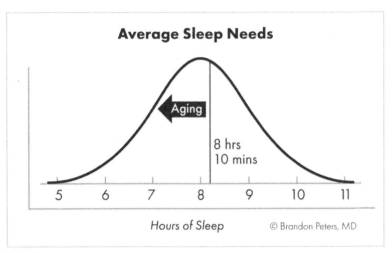

Average Sleep Needs

Aging

8 hrs
10 mins

5   6   7   8   9   10   11

Hours of Sleep   © Brandon Peters, MD

Figure 5

a 7-hour sleep need, you will experience 2 hours of insomnia (at the beginning or in the middle of the night). In some cases, it's not insomnia, it's math. You just can't sleep that much! The difference between the amount of time you are able to sleep and the amount of time you are spending in bed will be made up with time spent awake. Even someone with a normal sleep ability would experience this. The average sleep need beyond 65 years of age is estimated to be 7 to 8 hours. Part of solving insomnia is discovering your sleep need, at your current stage of life, and adjusting your time in bed to better match this ability.

> *The average sleep need beyond 65 years of age is estimated to be 7 to 8 hours.*

"It's not insomnia, it's math."

What Is Insomnia? Discovering the Causes of Insomnia

Insomnia is defined as difficulty falling asleep or difficulty returning to sleep after nighttime awakenings. It is associated with daytime complaints of fatigue, tiredness, low energy, and exhaustion. Its occurrence can be understood by reviewing the model for insomnia originally developed by Arthur Spielman, PhD (see Figure 6).

Based on this model, the onset of insomnia is dependent on predisposing factors. Some people always sleep great, while others are more likely to develop insomnia. This is based on genetic factors (insomnia often runs in families), the presence of other sleep disorders, psychiatric conditions like anxiety or depression, and chronic pain. It may depend on an underlying difference in chemistry within the brain.

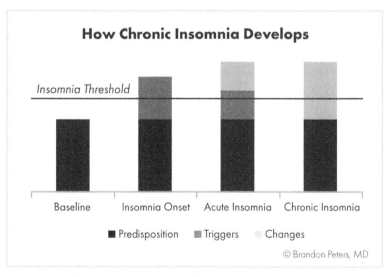

Figure 6: Adapted from Spielman AJ, Caruso L, Glovinsky PB. "A behavioral perspective on insomnia." *Psychiatr Clin North Am* 1987; 10:541–553.

Typically, insomnia first manifests due to precipitating factors or triggers. These can include environmental factors: an uncomfortable bed, noise, light, and temperature. Moreover, psychological or psychosocial factors may trigger insomnia, including stress from work, a divorce, or bereavement. If these triggers come and go, the insomnia resolves. However, sometimes changes develop that cause chronic insomnia to occur.

Chronic insomnia is defined as insomnia that occurs at least 3 nights per week and has lasted for at least 3 months. It may last for years or even decades. It is often due to changes or factors that have perpetuated the condition. For example, the pattern of sleep may change: going to bed early, staying in bed late into the morning, or taking naps. The basic sleep need may be exceeded by too much time spent in bed. This can thin out sleep and worsen its quality. It can also condition us to associate the bed with wakefulness. Sometimes our relationship to sleep can change: sleep becomes stressful, a source of anxiety, anger, and frustration. None of these feelings are conducive to sleep. Any can make it harder to sleep at night. Untreated sleep disorders can also cause insomnia to persist.

No matter the causes of prolonged insomnia, these can be identified and defused as part of insomnia treatment. This can reset your sleep to normal in a matter of weeks. In addition, you will learn a set of skills that can be applied should you experience an episode of insomnia in the future. This program can provide lasting change to aid your sleep for the rest of your life.

Introduction to the Sleep Log

The first task is to start by documenting your current sleep pattern. This is meant to be reflective and instructive. By establishing a baseline, you can begin to make targeted changes to help resolve your insomnia. It will help you to identify what you are doing well and may highlight some areas for improvement.

It is recommended that you document your sleep habits using the provided sleep logs (see p. 141). This self-reported form will help you to gauge your response to therapy as it evolves over the course of the program. Alternatively, you can consider the use of the free CBT-I Coach app available from the U.S. Department of Veterans Affairs. Fitness and activity trackers may also be used as an adjunct to this program, though the data may not be 100 percent accurate.

Do not become overly concerned about monitoring your sleep to complete the sleep log. It should be a rough assessment of your sleep, not a precise measurement. It is not about accuracy and you should not watch the clock at night to document the numbers.

You may be terrible at reporting this information, but you will be the constant all along as the logs are completed. If you overestimate, or underreport, it is likely that you will be somewhat consistent. Ultimately, it is about your experience of sleep—and its improvements—that matters in the end.

Complete the sleep log summary daily in the morning upon awakening. Start by listing any sleep aids (including prescription or over-the-counter medications) that you took before bedtime or in the night. Note when you crawled into bed and what time you turned out the lights to go to sleep (if it was later). Document how long it took you to fall asleep (again, use your best estimate: was it 5 minutes or 2 hours?). Note how many times you woke in the night, and how much time was spent awake. It does not matter when you woke up, but it is helpful to know roughly how much time was spent awake in the course of the night. Report what time you finally woke for the day and when you got out of bed (if it was later). Consider how long you felt like you slept and give your sleep a subjective quality rating. If you took a nap the day preceding the night's sleep, make a note of it, as it could impact your sleep. Finally, make a note of any other events, activities, or substance use (caffeine or alcohol) that may have either helped or harmed your ability to sleep.

Make an effort to complete the sleep log each morning. If you fail to do this, it may delay your progress. This first week it is about establishing your baseline. If you sleep poorly, that's okay, as it will only get better from here.

Setting Program Goals

Before embarking on this program, take a moment to reflect on what you hope to accomplish and how you shall measure personal success. In 6 weeks, you will be done with the program: How do you hope to sleep? Do you want to discontinue the use of a sleep aid? What will indicate you need further help or even a sleep study? The goal is to sleep normally without the use of medications, so keep this week's reading in mind as you set about the work ahead. Consider these goals and add the milestones you seek to meet:

☐ Discontinue Sleep Aids

☐ Time to Fall Asleep Initially: _____ (minutes)

☐ Decrease Wakefulness after Sleep Onset

☐ Total Sleep Time: _____ (hours)

☐ Sleep Timing:

    ☐ Goal Wake Time: _____

    ☐ Goal Bedtime: _____

☐ Improve Daytime Function

☐ Consider a Sleep Evaluation or Study If Symptoms Persist

These program goals will guide us through the weeks and they will be revisited at the end of the program to ensure its success. Changes will unfold over weeks and months. Progress may be incremental. There may be weeks of significant strides, a revelatory turning point when everything comes together, and even some setbacks. Fortunately, most people will ultimately be able to reach these long-term goals.

Conclusion

This week we have reviewed other medical and psychiatric conditions that may contribute to insomnia and interfere with program success. We have started to learn about the basics of normal sleep, sleep needs, and the potential causes of insomnia. We have reviewed how to use a sleep log to track sleep patterns over the course of the program. We have also established the ultimate goals that we will meet upon successful completion of the program. Now focus on the following weekly goals and return to this text in 1 week with your first completed sleep log.

Week 1 Goals:

- Start keeping a sleep log (p. 141).
- Try to observe a fixed wake time by getting up at the same time every day.
- Get 15 to 30 minutes of morning sunlight upon awakening (or at sunrise).

Note: After your first week of keeping a sleep log, return to this text and begin the next book chapter.

Sleep Consolidation and CBT-I

Reflection: Baseline Sleep
Education: How to Enhance Sleep
Goal Setting: Sleep Consolidation

Learning Objectives:

- Review your baseline sleep log to begin to recognize patterns and contributors to insomnia and identify initial targets for change.
- Discover ways to enhance sleep quality, including the important contributions of the sleep drive and circadian rhythm.
- Learn about the effectiveness and components of the cognitive behavioral therapy for insomnia (CBT-I) program, including:

sleep consolidation, stimulus control, buffer zone, scheduled worry time, and relaxation training.

- Identify activities to promote wakefulness and to aid the transition to sleep.
- Set goals for the first week of sleep consolidation.

How to Analyze a Sleep Log

 The first order of business in returning to the program's education component each week is to reflect on how you did by reviewing the documentation of your sleep log.

REALITY CHECK

Last week's primary goal, to document your baseline sleep habits, should have been easily achieved. If you did not do it, now is the time to commit yourself more fully to the program's requirements—and you may consider delaying the next phase until you have completed this important documentation.

Take a moment to glance over your completed sleep log. How did you do in completing it? Did you manage to fill in all the boxes? Were there any that you left blank that you can complete now? These data are most helpful if you provide a complete accounting of your experiences, but don't let this become a source of anxious preoccupation at night. These are meant to be estimates, not exact numbers.

Now consider how well (or how poorly) you slept each night and over the week:

- How often did you need to use your sleeping pills?
- Did your bedtime vary?
- How much time was spent falling asleep at the beginning of the night?
- Did you wake frequently or spend prolonged periods awake during the night?
- Was there any clear pattern? For example, was a night or two of particularly bad sleep followed by a night of improved sleep?
- Was your wake time regular and fixed (as was intended) or did you let it vary depending on how the night had gone?
- Did you take naps to make up for poor sleep—and was there an impact on your next night's sleep?
- On average, how many hours were spent in bed and how much time in total were you actually sleeping?
- Did you notice any difference in how you felt as you started to get sunlight exposure each morning?

After reflecting on your baseline sleep, you may feel despondent in how poorly you are sleeping. Turn this on its head: the worse you slept this week, the more improvement you can potentially have as part of this program! Don't lose hope—it gets better from here. At the end of this chapter, specific goals will be set for the week ahead. Now you can start to learn how to enhance the quality of sleep at night.

How Sleep Is Regulated

Let us consider how natural processes in your body that occur without fail can help you to sleep better. Good sleep is dependent on two processes: the *homeostatic sleep drive* and the *circadian alerting rhythm*. Understanding these contributors to sleep and wakefulness can help us to make changes to improve the quality of our sleep.

Homeostatic sleep drive is sometimes called sleep load or sleep debt. It is the fact that the longer you stay awake, the sleepier you will become. As an example, if you were kept awake for 30 hours, at the end of that time you would feel very sleepy, fall asleep very quickly, sleep deeply, and you might even sleep longer than usual. This is due to the accumulation of chemicals within the brain that contribute to sleepiness.

Adenosine is the most important chemical that works as a sleep signal. It is created as a normal part of energy metabolism in the body. Every cell in the body uses adenosine triphosphate (ATP) as its energy source: the phosphate bonds are broken one by one and the power stored in those bonds powers the cell. Eventually, once all of the three phosphate atoms are removed, adenosine is left over. The longer we stay awake, the more energy our brain uses, and the more that adenosine accumulates and makes us feel sleepy.

There is no way to break this system: your body will unfailingly use ATP as its energy source and as it is used in the brain, a chemical that contributes to sleepiness will build up. There may be individual variation in how quickly adenosine accumulates or, more likely, how efficiently it is removed. There may be other brain chemicals at play as well. For example, keep in mind that anxiety may easily override any signal for sleepiness. This becomes important as we consider the necessity of relaxing in the hour before going to sleep and, if sleep is becoming difficult, resetting ourselves by getting up and returning to bed later when the anxiety has subsided.

The levels of adenosine are lowest in the morning and build gradually with wakefulness (see Figure 7). The levels are highest in the hours preceding sleep onset. Sleep is, at least in part, a process of clearing away these chemicals. There is evidence that something called the **glymphatic system** exists to flush these chemicals from the brain's tissues during sleep. If we only sleep half a night, there is insufficient time to remove adenosine and we wake feeling sleepy. If we take a prolonged nap in the afternoon or evening, the chemical will be partially cleared and we may have more trouble falling asleep that night. If we sleep in one morning, we may not have sufficient time to build a strong drive for sleep by

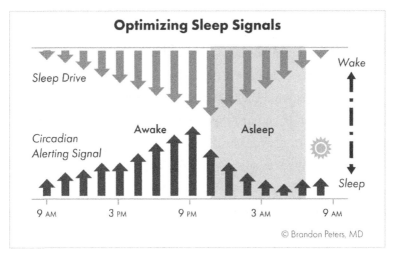

Figure 7: Adapted from Borbély AA. "A two process model of sleep regulation." *Hum Neurobiol* 1982;1:195–204.

> **Insomnia is a deflated balloon.**

our normal bedtime due to the shortened time spent awake during the day.

Imagine that strengthening the drive for sleep is like filling up a balloon with sleepiness: the longer you are awake, the fuller the balloon becomes, but sleep will slowly empty it. This fact can be used to our advantage. Insomnia is a deflated balloon. If you wake towards morning, it may be harder to get back to sleep because the balloon is almost empty. Sleeping in can also shorten the time we have during the day to fill the balloon. By delaying our bedtime while keeping the wake time fixed, as occurs through the process of **sleep consolidation**, we can fill the balloon more, making the sleep drive stronger. We will begin this process this week to enhance your natural ability to sleep.

It is important to understand that there are also substances we consume that can block or enhance the effects of adenosine. **Caffeine** blocks this sleepy signal and makes us feel more awake. It makes it harder to fall asleep, increases light sleep (stages 1 and 2), and decreases total sleep time, stage 3, and REM sleep. It can be important to avoid the use of caffeine for at least 4 to 6 hours before bedtime. If you are especially sensitive, you may need to consider abstaining even earlier, such as after noon.

Alcohol enhances adenosine levels and we can become sleepy (and even pass out) if we drink too much. Traditionally (when sleeping pills were not available), alcohol was relied on as a sleep aid, with older generations having a "nightcap," or alcoholic drink, before going to bed. It does make it transiently easier to fall asleep, but the effects are short-lived. Alcohol wears off quickly, with one drink often metabolized in an hour or two, and this will fragment sleep. Alcohol is known to shorten REM sleep. It may cause airway muscle relaxation and worsen sleep apnea, leading to further awakenings. It is thus not a good sleep aid. It should be avoided several hours before going to sleep.

The complement to sleep drive is the **circadian alerting signal**. It counteracts or balances the signal for sleepiness. It is relatively weak in the morning: it doesn't have much work to do. It starts to build gradually and becomes very strong in the evening, when we don't feel too sleepy even though it's at the end of the day (see Figure 7). It falls off very quickly at sleep onset and stays low overnight.

There is a natural lull in the circadian alerting signal in the afternoon—often around 1:00 to 3:00 p.m.—that correlates with an increased desire for sleep. Everyone is more likely to feel sleepy then, especially after inadequate hours of (or poor quality) sleep. People think it relates to eating a heavy lunch, but it does not; you eat dinner and you are not particularly sleepy afterwards. It has everything to do with the circadian rhythm. Societies have adopted social practices that encourage caffeine consumption (often coffee or tea) with an afternoon break or a nap (especially in cultures closer to the equator) at that time. Even if we don't take a nap or have a coffee, we begin to wake more in the subsequent hours as the circadian alerting signal ramps up into the late afternoon and early evening.

The timing of the circadian (Latin for "near day") system is written into our genetics. If isolated in a cave, a constant environment of light and darkness, we would still sleep about 8 hours and be awake about 16 hours—but not exactly. Our internal clock is usually off a little, and in most people it runs about 24½ hours. This means that in the cave we would want to go to bed and wake 30 minutes later every day without realizing it. The thing that keeps us on track, that resets our clock, is exposure to morning sunlight upon awakening. This helps to align our natural tendency towards sleep to the patterns of light and darkness in our environment.

The central control of the body's circadian rhythms is within the hypothalamus, located in a part of the brain called the suprachiasmatic nucleus (SCN) that sits near nerves that extend from the eyes. Light exposure changes these rhythms (see Figure 8). The closer the light exposure occurs to our minimum core body temperature (Tmin), the more powerful its effects. This Tmin occurs about 2 hours before our natural waking time. If light exposure occurs after it, the timing of sleep advances earlier (with a sleep onset and wake time happening earlier). If light exposure occurs right before the Tmin, the timing of sleep may delay later. This has important consequences when considering the effects of artificial light.

It may be best to avoid blue light exposure from artificial sources preceding bedtime. In particular, smartphones, computers, and tablets may be especially impactful, as the device screens are positioned relatively close to the eyes. A television across the room may not have the same impact. Though the levels of screen light may be modest, some individuals (especially night owls) may be particularly sensitive. If you believe it impacts your sleep, use of artificial light should be minimized in the 1 to 2 hours before bedtime. It may also be possible to switch some electronic devices to a "night mode," which reduces the blue spectrum of

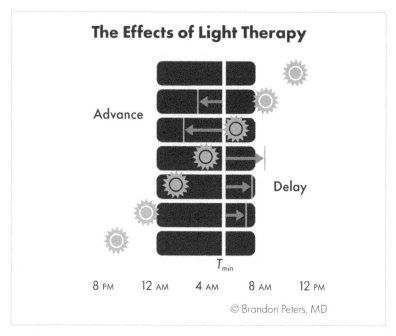

Figure 8

light. Some people even use special amber-colored screen covers or orange-lensed glasses (often called "blue blockers") that filter out the blue light.

Finally, it may be possible to counteract these evening effects of artificial light by simply getting exposed to natural light upon awakening. This can be highly effective. Ideally, the light exposure should occur for at least 15 minutes immediately upon awakening (or right after sunrise). Sun is best. Get outside and look towards the sun without a hat, visor, or sunglasses. You can read, go for a walk, eat breakfast, or even play on your phone while enjoying the light. Morning sunlight enhances our ability to fall asleep and serves as a strong signal for wakefulness, initiating the circadian alerting signal. This may be especially important in certain circadian rhythm sleep disorders. If morning sunlight cannot be naturally obtained, the use of a 10,000-lux light box may be a helpful substitute. Fixing the wake time each morning, no matter how poor sleep has been and even on weekends or days off, also helps to reinforce these patterns.

Night Owls and Morning Larks: Circadian Disorders

The timing of sleep can be off in specific circadian rhythm disorders (see Figure 9). **Delayed sleep phase syndrome** is typified by night owls who struggle to get to sleep before midnight and also have difficulty waking early. It affects about 10 percent of the population and begins in adolescence but may persist throughout life.

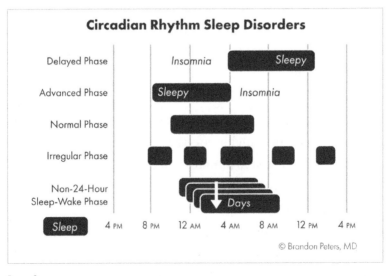

Figure 9

These individuals often lie awake for hours if they try to go to bed earlier, and may not feel fully awake until several hours into the day. Many experience extreme sleep deprivation and may sleep in on weekends or days off to catch up on lost sleep.

Other circadian disorders occur less often. **Advanced sleep phase syndrome** is the opposite of delayed sleep phase syndrome, with evening sleepiness and early morning awakenings. It may affect about 1 percent of people. It is important to note that early morning awakenings may also occur due to sleep apnea and may be associated with depression. An **irregular sleep-wake rhythm** occurs among the elderly with dementing illnesses like Alzheimer's disease. They lose the system controlling the ability to get a continuous period of sleep at night. As a result, they have short periods of sleep (typically lasting 1 to 2 hours) and wakefulness scattered throughout the 24-hour day. Though people with insomnia may also wake frequently during the night, it is unlikely that a developing dementia is a cause of the disorder.

Finally, totally blind people who completely lack light perception (either acquired or from birth) may experience **Non-24**. This was previously called having a free-running circadian rhythm. They are dependent on their internal clock to establish sleep-wake patterns without perceiving sunlight to reset it. It is almost like they are living in that constant cave environment. As previously mentioned, this internal clock is genetically programmed and is off a little each day, leading to a shifting pattern of insomnia and daytime sleepiness that typically unfolds over a few weeks among the blind. They often require the use of melatonin, taken hours before their desired bedtime, as an external signal for sleep.

Light exposure is especially important for management of insomnia among sighted individuals with circadian rhythm disorders, especially delayed sleep phase syndrome.

Introduction to CBT-I Concepts

Cognitive behavioral therapy for insomnia (CBT-I) is typically structured as a 6-week treatment program that can help to relieve chronic insomnia. CBT-I may be effectively conducted through one-on-one sessions with a provider, in group classes, or via self-directed programs outlined in books or provided online. It is a scientifically proven, goal-directed therapy that is usually driven by data collected with sleep logs. Skills are learned to prevent future relapses of chronic insomnia. It is more than just basic sleep advice. The treatment components of CBT-I include:

Sleep Consolidation

This is the first major change as part of a CBT-I program. It involves using your baseline sleep pattern obtained during the first week to make adjustments to your bedtime and wake time to better reflect your natural ability to sleep and actual sleep needs (see Figure 10). Prior to sleep consolidation, you may have difficulty falling asleep and spend prolonged periods awake in the night, especially after waking towards morning. Though 8 hours may be spent in bed, only 6 hours of sleep may be achieved. Sleep consolidation may require delaying your bedtime by several hours, or waking slightly earlier, to build the sleep drive and enhance your ability to sleep. We shall review your actual schedule and required adjustment towards the end of this chapter. Often people start

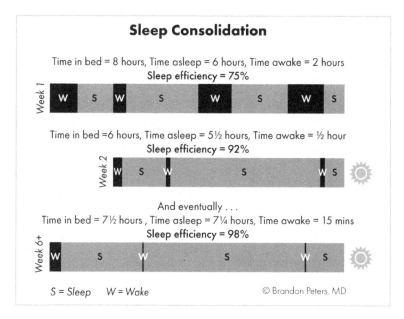

Figure 10

spending too much time in bed when they are sleeping poorly and this can worsen insomnia. Spending less time in bed often results in a deeper, higher-quality sleep with fewer awakenings. Once sleep efficiency (the total amount of sleep divided by the total amount of time in bed) improves, the period of time in bed is extended to obtain adequate hours of sleep to feel rested without insomnia recurring. This gradual adjustment helps to find your optimal sleep pattern to meet your sleep needs and fully eliminate insomnia.

Stimulus Control

This is breaking the association between the bed and wakefulness. With insomnia, conditioning can occur that may cause anxiety and wakefulness to be associated with our sleep environment. This may exacerbate difficulty sleeping. The bed is a place for sleep. Keep your phone in the kitchen to charge overnight. Ideally, don't watch TV in bed before turning out the lights. If you struggle to fall asleep, you may begin to associate the bed not just with wakefulness, but also with anxiety, frustration, or anger. None of these feelings are conducive to sleep. You may even dread going to bed, or develop an aversion to your bed or bedroom. It becomes a place of struggle and torment; you may never know what the night will bring. This must be reset with more positive associations and experiences that consistently result in a favorable transition to sleep. This conditioning is strengthened by going to bed and turning the lights out immediately, reserving the bed only for sleep and sex, getting out of bed if awake more than 15 to 20 minutes in the night, and getting up immediately upon awakening in the morning.

> *The bed is a place for sleep.*

Buffer Zone

This is preserving time at the end of the day to relax and unwind before going to bed. By preparing the body and mind to sleep with an orderly transition, sleep will more easily come. Our bodies respond best to regular patterns. Ideally, 30 to 60 minutes are spent in quiet activities such as reading, watching TV or a movie, or listening to music before going to bed. Avoid doing these activities in bed, but choose another place to relax. Reviewing a list of suggestions may be helpful (see pp. 40–44).

Scheduled Worry Time

This is scheduling a time in the day to manage stressors by writing them down and creating an action plan to address them in order to relieve anxiety or mind-racing at night. This will be reviewed during Week 4 of the program.

Relaxation Techniques

The use of breathing techniques, progressive muscle relaxation, guided imagery, and mindfulness may help to distract a busy mind at night and ease the transition to sleep. This will also be reviewed during Week 4 of the program.

Other factors that contribute to insomnia can also be addressed as needed. Caffeine or alcohol use, exposure to artificial light at night, eating too close to bedtime, a disruptive sleep environment, alarm clock checking, poor sleep in your spouse or children, and other factors may play a role. Consider your situation and whether adjustments should be made to obtain relief.

Does CBT-I Work?

Research consistently demonstrates that CBT-I is highly effective. From 2013 to 2016, 199 people participated in my clinic-based program. The average age was 61 years and 63 percent of the patients were women. Just over 77 percent were using sleeping pills when they started the program, but they weren't sleeping that well. By the end of the program, the time it took to fall asleep had improved from 45.2 minutes to 22.2 minutes. The time spent awake in the night, after falling asleep, decreased from 46.1 to 27.3 minutes. The average total number of hours of sleep per night also increased.

It is important to recognize that sleep apnea was extremely common in this group: it was diagnosed in 74 percent and another 16 percent were suspected of having the condition based on their symptoms and anatomy. Sleep apnea is associated with snoring, daytime sleepiness, teeth grinding, and getting up to urinate at night. Therefore, as already discussed in Week 1 and to be further revisited in Week 5, a sleep study may be an important part of your treatment program, especially if you have persistent night-time awakenings after your insomnia has improved.

Identifying Ways to Promote Sleep and Wakefulness

Many people respond with disbelief (it's coming!) when considering how late they must stay up the first week of sleep consolidation. It may make you feel anxious. When considering a later bedtime, you may wonder, "What am I going to do until *then*?" Surprisingly, by the end of the week, you may actually find it difficult to stay awake until your goal bedtime. How is that for a reversal!

Fortunately, here (starting on p. 40) you will find a long list of possible activities to consider. You will want to identify things to do during the last hour of the day as you transition to sleep as part of your buffer zone. Put a checkmark in the column labeled "Get Sleepy." These should be relaxing, preparing your body and mind for the transition to sleep. These same activities may be appropriate if you wake in the night and get out of bed as you observe stimulus control, hoping to get sleepy with the activity to return to bed.

If you feel *too sleepy* prior to your bedtime, or perhaps in mid-afternoon, you may also need ideas to keep yourself awake. Avoid taking naps to enhance your sleep at night. For these wake-promoting activities, put a checkmark in the column labeled "Stay Awake." These activities often include cleaning, sorting, and organizing—physically moving to keep yourself awake. As you become more sleepy through the week, avoid any activities in which it would be dangerous to fall asleep (especially driving drowsy). Rest assured: by the end of the first week, your insomnia will be improved, and your house will be cleaner and more organized than it has been in months!

The following list of activities is organized for you. It starts with activities that you may find relaxing, for use in the hour before going to bed or in the night. It transitions to those that may be more stimulating and may help to keep you awake if you are feeling too sleepy. Finally, it ends with blanks to add your own ideas. Some suggestions may focus on yourself, and others may be directed toward others. You will notice the following themes or categories of activities are present:

- Relaxation
- Hobbies/Games
- Health/Self-Help
- Spiritual
- Family/Relationship
- Planning/Shopping
- Organization/Sorting
- Cleaning
- Educational/Professional
- Financial

Carefully review the list, identifying activities for each scenario described above—both to get sleepy and to stay awake. Some activities may be appropriate for either category. If the idea is not applicable to you, leave it blank and move to the next one.

If at any point this week you need suggestions for how to relax before bed, or what to do if you are feeling too sleepy, come back to the list and select your favorite task. Complete this section now.

Activity	Stay Awake	Get Sleepy
Read a book for pleasure.	☐	☐
Read low-stress (or old) articles in the newspaper or online.	☐	☐
Read a magazine or trade journal.	☐	☐
Look through catalogs or advertisements.	☐	☐
Watch a favorite movie that is not too stimulating.	☐	☐
Watch television shows that you have seen before.	☐	☐
Watch repetitive television like infomercials, CNN, C-SPAN, or The Weather Channel.	☐	☐
Listen to slow, relaxing, or instrumental music.	☐	☐
Spend time on your favorite hobby.	☐	☐
Assemble photo albums or scrapbooks.	☐	☐
Work on crafts or handiwork like quilting, embroidery, crocheting, or knitting.	☐	☐
Complete puzzles like crosswords, word search, or sudoku.	☐	☐
Play solitaire on your computer or with a deck of cards.	☐	☐
Play a board game.	☐	☐

Put together a puzzle.	☐	☐
Practice a musical instrument.	☐	☐
Take a bath or long shower.	☐	☐
Give yourself a pedicure, manicure, or facial.	☐	☐
Floss your teeth and gums.	☐	☐
Choose clothes that you can wear the next day.	☐	☐
Have a light snack or a small drink (i.e., water, warm milk).	☐	☐
Groom or play with your pets.	☐	☐
Exercise.	☐	☐
Do some stretching or practice yoga.	☐	☐
Go for a walk alone, with family or friends, or with your dog.	☐	☐
Take a bicycle ride.	☐	☐
Go for a swim.	☐	☐
Go to the gym.	☐	☐
Use your exercise equipment at home.	☐	☐
Practice your favorite sport.	☐	☐
Dance to your favorite music.	☐	☐
If awake too early, watch the sunrise.	☐	☐
Go to a coffee shop.	☐	☐
Write a short story or poem based on a favorite memory.	☐	☐
Write in your journal.	☐	☐
Write down or review your list of thoughts as part of scheduled worry time.	☐	☐
Meditate or pray.	☐	☐
Participate in a church or community project.	☐	☐
Find a local organization in need and volunteer.	☐	☐
Talk to your spouse or children.	☐	☐

Telephone acquaintances who live in other time zones.	☐	☐
Update your address book on paper or online.	☐	☐
Add birthdays to a paper calendar.	☐	☐
Send cards for upcoming birthdays, anniversaries, or holidays.	☐	☐
Send emails to friends and family.	☐	☐
Write personal thank-you, get well soon, and sympathy notes.	☐	☐
Work on the family tree.	☐	☐
Spend time interacting via social media (Facebook, Twitter, Pinterest, Instagram, etc.).	☐	☐
Surf the internet.	☐	☐
Make gifts for friends.	☐	☐
Shop for holiday, birthday, wedding, or baby gifts online.	☐	☐
Shop online extravagantly and then empty the shopping cart.	☐	☐
Explore an online auction site like eBay for your favorite items.	☐	☐
Do research for major purchases like houses, cars, or appliances.	☐	☐
Create a list of materials needed for a project around the house.	☐	☐
Make a detailed menu and ingredient list for the week's meals.	☐	☐
Put together a grocery shopping list for the upcoming week.	☐	☐
Go to the grocery store or run other errands.	☐	☐
Make your lunch.	☐	☐
Prepare meals for the week in advance.	☐	☐
Marinate or start to prepare food for the following day.	☐	☐

Do some baking or make a dessert.	☐	☐
Plan the layout of your garden.	☐	☐
Review your to-do list for the day or the week.	☐	☐
Create a list of activities you would enjoy doing on weekends or while on vacation.	☐	☐
Set up a pillbox with medications for the week.	☐	☐
Sort through boxes stored in closets, the attic, the garage, or under beds.	☐	☐
Clean out the kitchen pantry and identify food that should be disposed of or could be donated.	☐	☐
Organize collections of items (books, recipes, photos, old letters, coins, stamps, wine, albums, CDs, DVDs, board games, sheet music, or other things) and choose some to donate or sell if you no longer enjoy them.	☐	☐
Try on clothes and identify items that could go to charity or be sold.	☐	☐
Go through the children's toys or clothes and choose things to get rid of.	☐	☐
Select some drawers or cupboards to clean out in the desk, kitchen, or bathroom.	☐	☐
Remove clutter from tables, countertops, or your desk.	☐	☐
Do the dishes and wipe down the counters.	☐	☐
Wash the dishes in the china cabinet.	☐	☐
Sweep or mop the kitchen floor.	☐	☐
Clean out the refrigerator.	☐	☐
Clean the bathroom.	☐	☐
Do the laundry.	☐	☐
Fold clothes and put them away.	☐	☐
Polish your shoes, iron, or mend clothing.	☐	☐
Make your bed and tidy in your bedroom.	☐	☐

Decorate for an upcoming holiday.	☐	☐
Open or close the curtains and blinds in the house.	☐	☐
Sweep your sidewalk or steps or shovel snow.	☐	☐
Do some light gardening and yard work or water the houseplants.	☐	☐
Complete maintenance or a household project.	☐	☐
Clear out your email inbox.	☐	☐
Organize, back up, or (if unwanted) delete your computer files.	☐	☐
Practice or learn a new skill or language.	☐	☐
Go to the library and research a new topic of interest.	☐	☐
Get a travel or history book and learn about your favorite city.	☐	☐
Plan an upcoming or dream vacation.	☐	☐
Get ready for work early.	☐	☐
Open mail and sort out junk mail and bills (but avoid paying bills).	☐	☐
Clear out old stored tax records.	☐	☐
Organize all your bills, receipts, coupons, and warranty information.	☐	☐
Gather old bills, statements, and documents and shred them.	☐	☐
Start a budget for your family on a spreadsheet or in a notebook.	☐	☐
	☐	☐
	☐	☐
	☐	☐
	☐	☐
	☐	☐
	☐	☐

Beginning the Process of Change

Now that you have reflected on your baseline sleep log, learned about ways to enhance your natural ability to sleep, been introduced to some of the basic concepts of CBT-I, and identified activities to help you to transition to sleep or to stay awake, it is time to begin the process of change. Change is exciting, but it can also be a little intimidating.

Know that this upcoming week can be a tough one. As part of sleep consolidation, you may become slightly sleep deprived. People often feel more irritable, with increased problems with thinking (especially affecting concentration and short-term memory) and mood. Pain may be increased. These effects are quickly reversed, even after just one night of recovery sleep. Be cautious with driving this week: don't drive if you feel too sleepy. Let others know that this may be a difficult week for you. Don't make any major life decisions. Every other symptom is transient and will resolve gradually as your sleep is enhanced. Understand that you are likely to feel very sleepy at times, but the more you are able to adhere to these recommendations, the sooner you can begin to ease up on the demands. Insomnia may not relent in the first few nights, but by the end of the first week, you will recognize the improvements that are starting to occur.

Consolidating Sleep to Improve Insomnia

 Take a moment to review your baseline sleep log from last week. The sleep log is your means to track the changes and improvement you experience over the course of the program. As you begin to learn about ways to enhance

> You can't set an alarm to fall asleep, but you can set an alarm to wake up.

your ability to sleep, you will recognize areas for improvement. This week will focus on adjusting your time in bed to better reflect your current ability to sleep and sleep needs.

When you look at your sleep log from last week, what is the average time that you naturally wake up? Start by focusing here: you can't set an alarm to fall asleep, but you can set an alarm to wake up. Select a wake time that you can adhere to each and every day of this next week. You will get up at this time, no matter how good or bad the night is. You will get up at this time on days off. If you would like to be getting up earlier than the recent average, this can be a longer-term goal with a gradual adjustment, but start where you are. Fix your wake time and commit to setting a daily alarm and getting 15 to 30 minutes of sunlight immediately upon awakening.

Do not check the clock at night (cover or turn the alarm clock after setting it and put away other timepieces like watches and phones). Checking the time at night can provoke thinking ("How long have I slept?" or "How long do I have left to sleep?") and negative emotions like anxiety, frustration, or anger. If you wake up and do not hear your alarm, it is not time to get up; roll over and try to go back to sleep.

Take a moment to estimate the number of hours that you are sleeping on average based on last week's sleep log. If a night is particularly bad, with little or no sleep obtained, you may want to ignore it as an outlier. Most people with insomnia average about 6 to 7 hours of sleep per night. If you feel like you are currently getting less sleep than this, use 6 hours as your minimum.

Now, it is possible to identify your bedtime by planning to spend only the number of hours in bed that you are actually sleeping. (Here is where the looks of shock and moments of protestation occur!) If you choose 7:00 a.m. as your wake time, and you are currently averaging 7 hours of sleep, you should select 12:00 a.m. as your goal bedtime for this week. Do not spend fewer than 6 hours of time in bed, no matter how little you feel you are sleeping on average. Determine your goal bedtime based on your wake time, working backwards from your goal wake time using your average total sleep time from last week. Plan to go to bed this week at this bedtime with the intent of immediately turning out the lights to go to sleep.

Now, take a deep breath. There are a few concerns that commonly come up at this point:

- You may wonder how you could possibly stay up that late (review your list of activities you just completed for ideas to stay awake). If you start to feel sleepy before your goal bedtime, get up, move around, and be more active. Don't fall asleep on the couch while you are waiting for your bedtime to come and really try hard to avoid going to bed earlier than your goal.

- Some worry about a "second wind" right before bedtime interfering with their ability to fall asleep. If you are not feeling sleepy, wait. The bedtime selected is a goal but not a deadline: if you are not feeling sleepy, continue to stay up doing something relaxing until you are. You want to go to bed when feeling drowsy or sleepy (not tired, fatigued, or exhausted) with heavy eyelids, a warm feeling in the body, and a strong desire for sleep.

- What if I stay up past my goal bedtime or wake too early? It is always okay to stay up later, or to get up earlier, than your goals as this will simply enhance your desire for sleep as you build the signal for sleepiness even stronger. If you wake before your alarm and can't get back to sleep, get up and see if there is enough time to relax and come back to bed. If it is close to morning and your goal wake time, you may just start your day a little earlier.

- Some worry that if they already spend hours awake at night with insomnia, reducing time in bed will reduce their sleep time even further. This concern does not persist beyond the first few nights: you will start to spend more of the time you are in bed actually sleeping. While feeling sleepy, avoid taking naps and don't go to bed too early (unless you absolutely hit a wall one night and simply must). Though you may not sleep through all of the time you are allowed in the first few nights, this gets better as the week progresses.

- What if you don't get enough sleep? You already don't get enough sleep. Particularly anxious people with insomnia even question, "Will I die?" Well, are you dead? People often go an entire night without sleep (think of resident doctors on call at the hospital). You will be able to function, even if not optimally, and you will get through your week. Sleep deprivation is not acutely harmful, assuming you don't drive drowsy. Muddle through the tough days and know it gets better.

- What if I wake up at night and can't get back to sleep? If by your estimate you are awake for longer than 15 minutes at night, get up and do something relaxing, and return to bed when you are feeling sleepy. This helps to recondition you and your association of the bed with sleep. It is acceptable to look at the time if you are out of bed on these occasions to determine if you will have enough time to get feeling sleepy, or if you should just be up for the day.

You will discover, as you have for years, that you can function on a reduced total sleep time for a week. The rewards of sleep consolidation will quickly become apparent as insomnia relents and then the pressure will be eased.

By the end of the week, if you can stick to your goals, you will be falling asleep faster and returning to sleep quicker if you wake in the night. Those participants who do the best are very strict with their schedule. The closer you can adhere to your goals, the better you will do. The sleep quality will be enhanced, with deeper, more restorative sleep, and insomnia will quickly fade away. You may not feel completely rested this week—and that is okay. Over the next several weeks the bedtime will be advanced earlier to replenish this lost sleep. Ultimately, you will get enough sleep and be sleeping normally, all in just a few short weeks.

Conclusion

This week we have reflected on your baseline sleep log, learned about ways to enhance your natural ability to sleep through the homeostatic sleep drive and circadian alerting signal. We have identified the effects of caffeine and alcohol on sleep and introduced some of the basic concepts of CBT-I. We have identified activities to help you to transition to sleep or to stay awake. Finally, we have set and committed to the initial goals to begin sleep consolidation. Focus on these weekly goals and return to this text in 1 week with your completed sleep log.

Week 2 Goals:

- Continue keeping a sleep log (p. 141) to track your progress.
- Observe a fixed wake time by getting up at the same time every day with an alarm clock. Set the alarm clock for a goal wake time of _____.
- Do not check the clock at night. Set the alarm and turn or cover it at night to avoid clock checking.
- Get 15 to 30 minutes of morning sunlight upon awakening (or at sunrise).
- Avoid taking naps unless required for safety (and keep them brief if needed).
- Goal bedtime at _____ with lights out immediately. Spend 60 minutes relaxing before bedtime (using list for ideas). If necessary, stay up later until feeling sleepy.
- If awake for more than 15 minutes at night, by your estimate, get up and go to another room and do something relaxing until feeling sleepy and then come back to bed.
- Continue to use sleeping pills as you normally would.

Note: After your first week of sleep consolidation, return to this text and begin the next book chapter.

Sleep Extension and Conditioning

Reflection: Response to Consolidation
Education: Conditioning and Sleeping Pills
Goal Setting: Sleep Extension

Learning Objectives:

- Review your current sleep log to assess response to sleep consolidation and identify areas requiring improved adherence.
- Learn about the importance of improving conditioning and sleep associations by observing stimulus control.
- Discover ways to stay awake until your goal bedtime and how to enjoy your mornings.

- Understand the profiles of common sleeping pills, potential short- and long-term side effects, and the optimal plan for supervised tapering.
- Learn how to calculate sleep efficiency and use this information to begin the process of sleep extension.
- Set goals for the first week of sleep extension.

Assessing Changes after Sleep Consolidation

It is time again to review last week's sleep log. If you were successfully able to adhere to your goals from last week, you may have noted some significant changes as the week unfolded. Let's take a moment to reflect on how you did.

REALITY CHECK

Remind yourself of your goals from Week 2 as you review the sleep log. Take a highlighter and identify places where you may have strayed: either going to bed too early, staying in bed too late, or taking naps. If you really struggled to adhere to the recommendations set forth, consider whether you should try again this week before proceeding to make further changes. You are building a set of skills, and you want to ensure that you start with a solid foundation.

There are a few possible outcomes from the first week of sleep consolidation. Some people very strictly adhere to the recommendations, keeping to their goal bedtimes and wake times with an almost military-like precision. Generally, these people begin to quickly notice changes in their ability to fall asleep and to get back to sleep more easily after waking in the night (though the awakenings themselves may still persist). The sleep quality gradually increases. Within a few days, and certainly by the end of the week, insomnia begins to relent. There may be an occasional setback, but the trend is to the good. The total amount of sleep may be inadequate, leading to increasing daytime sleepiness, and this is why it next proves necessary to begin the process of sleep extension. These adjustments will be made based on the calculation of sleep efficiency, which will be introduced later in this chapter.

Another possibility is that the outcome of the week was less than desirable. There may have been minimal or no improvement. Some people even notice that their ability to sleep takes a significant step backwards. There are a few reasons this may occur. First, remember that underlying medical (e.g., sleep apnea, fibromyalgia) and psychiatric conditions (e.g., anxiety) may reduce the tolerance to sleep consolidation. If needed, revisit these possible issues from Chapter 1. It is also possible that the changes this week unmasked a condition that may have been just below the surface. Rarely, sleep consolidation and progress in the program may be impossible until the associated condition is treated (see Chapter 5). It may be necessary to take a break or move on to other aspects of the program, such as relaxation techniques, before further attempting sleep consolidation. It is also possible that poor adherence to the goals undermined your ability to reap the benefits.

Imagine that the list of instructions outlined as Week 2's goals are a recipe for good sleep. If at the end of the week, you have not experienced a good outcome, you may consider questioning either the recipe or the cook. How carefully and closely did you follow the directions? If you were baking a cake, and instead of mixing in one-quarter teaspoon of salt, you opted to add one-quarter cup, you shouldn't be surprised if you don't like the taste of the final product. Similarly, if you are not fully satisfied with the improvements from this week's changes, consider how well you adhered to your goals. If you didn't consistently observe the recommendations, but fell into old habits, you are following your program, not this one. It is best to closely follow the recipe provided and trust that it can work for you. Recommit to these changes.

The most likely outcome lies somewhere between these two extremes: there were efforts to adhere to the recommendations, but these goals were not fully met. Be honest and determine where your strengths and weaknesses were in following the guidelines. Where did you stray? Were there barriers to your success? How can you help to resolve those issues so that you can be more successful this week? The closer you can follow the recipe, the better you will do. Fortunately, tonight is a new night, and you will have the chance to try to implement these strategies again.

Ultimately, the success of this week will be determined based on the sleep efficiency you attained, and this will guide the next steps that you shall take on this journey. There may also be a simple trick that could be useful to reset your sleep, especially if you have an occasional bad night, and chances are that you may have been imperfect in observing the recommendation.

Optimize Conditioning with Stimulus Control

One of the major impediments to successful sleep consolidation is committing oneself to the idea that if you are unable to sleep, you should get out of bed. Beyond the impacts of sleep deprivation associated with sleep consolidation, this is often the hardest part of an insomnia therapy program. The last thing you want to do if you are unable to sleep is to get out of bed; you just desperately want sleep to come, and you convince yourself that it is imminent, even if you lie awake for hours. Understanding the importance of this and how it impacts the conditioning associated with our ability to sleep may give you the motivation needed to finally commit to this change.

Let's take a moment to discuss a classic concept that is part of any basic introduction to general psychology course: conditioning. This is perhaps best remembered due to a Russian scientist named Ivan Pavlov and his famous dogs. In the 1890s, Pavlov did an experiment after he noticed his caged dogs would salivate upon seeing him walk into a room, even if they were not being fed. He wondered if they were unconsciously responding to the sight of him because they learned to associate his presence with food. He decided to test his theory.

Pavlov began to ring a bell when he fed his dogs. Over time, the dogs became conditioned to associate the sound of the bell with the presence of food. Ultimately, he was able to stimulate salivation just by ringing the bell, even with him out of sight and in the absence of food. The dogs had been trained to subconsciously associate the

If you are unable to sleep, you should get out of bed.

bell with food, and their bodies responded with salivation when hearing it. This is called a Pavlovian response—and this conditioning applies to insomnia, too.

In the context of insomnia, the stimulus and response differ, but understanding the potential relationship will empower you to make an extremely helpful change. When sleep becomes difficult, the bed is no longer a desired haven for rest sought at the end of a productive day. It becomes a place of torment. We learn to associate the bed (stimulus) not with sleep, but with insomnia (conditioned response). Therefore, the circumstances and environment associated with the onset of sleep become a signal to initiate anxiety and wakefulness. People with insomnia may approach bedtime with increasing dread as their ability to sleep spirals out of their control. Not surprisingly, they may actually find that they can sleep better elsewhere (like on vacation or at a hotel). This negative association has to be changed, the pattern broken, for insomnia to relent.

How can this be achieved? It is best accomplished through the practice of stimulus control. This means that you alter how you respond to the conditions until this relationship improves. You must learn to again associate the bed with sleep. For perfect conditioning, all wakefulness (and anxiety) should be removed from the bed. This is probably unrealistic, as it is normal to wake at night, but prolonged wakefulness should not be tolerated. Go to bed feeling very sleepy, so that you fall asleep faster. Upon awakening in the morning, immediately get up and start the day. Reserve the bed and bedroom for sleep and sex alone. If you are awake for a prolonged period in the night, you must get up.

As part of this, limit the time spent lying awake in bed to 15 to 20 minutes, by your estimate. Give yourself a chance to fall asleep (or to fall back asleep), but if it is not happening, simply get up. Use it as a chance to reset your relationship with the bed. Wrap yourself in a blanket, or throw on a robe, and remove yourself from your bedroom. Engage in a relaxing activity and return when you are feeling sleepy again. If once back in bed you again become stimulated, respond by again getting up and only returning to bed later when you are even more sleepy. Do this as often as is necessary. Over time, just like Pavlov's dogs, you will again learn to associate the bed with sleep.

It cannot be overstated how important it is to come to bed feeling sleepy. Do not go to bed just because it is a certain time. Listen to your body. Wait until you are feeling sleepy. You probably do not eat at a regimented time every day, though the regular timing of meals may reinforce the patterns of hunger. It would be absurd to sit at a dining table at a set time waiting for your appetite to come. Instead, you eat when you are hungry, even if it is slightly later or earlier than usual. Why would you similarly crawl into bed without feeling sleepy? Come to bed with a strong appetite for sleep and you will sleep better.

In all likelihood, observing stimulus control will become less and less frequent once you are able to strictly adhere to it. You may do it often early in the week, or early in the program, but after a while you can set it aside. If a bad night recurs, no matter what is the cause, rely on the skill to again reset your ability to get feeling sleepy and optimize the conditioning needed to associate the bed with sleep.

Improve Wakefulness and Enjoy Your Mornings

During this first week of sleep consolidation, you likely discovered what it means to be profoundly sleepy. You may have struggled to stay awake during specific times of the day or with certain passive activities. Who would have thought that after one short week you would transition from trouble going to sleep to struggling to stay awake until your goal bedtime? It may also have been difficult to force yourself out of the bed in the morning, which may be worsened if you are a night owl. These are two sides of the same coin: let's review some ways to optimize wakefulness and consider how to motivate getting up in the morning.

Reflect on how it feels to be sleepy and awake.

Recall what it has felt like this week to feel very sleepy and drowsy. These are distinct feelings from fatigue, tiredness, low energy, and exhaustion. Contrast this sleepiness with what it feels like to have optimal wakefulness and alertness. Take a moment to consider what other feelings or experiences—physical, mental, and emotional—are associated with these two states for you. (Continue to use sleepiness as your signal to go to bed, assuming you have reached your goal bedtime.) Think how mental clarity differs between these two states in regards to concentration, attention, and short-term memory as well as the impacts on productivity and proneness to errors. How does your mood change when you sleep well and feel alert? Rediscovering these feelings, especially after a long period in which the connection has been lost, can be a worthwhile exercise.

Identify the times and situations when you feel too sleepy.
If you struggled to avoid napping or dozing, going to bed too early, or sleeping in this past week, you may need help minimizing the impacts of sleepiness as you complete sleep extension over the next several weeks. Most people will feel especially sleepy certain times of the day, often in the midafternoon and late evening. Know when you are likely to feel sleepy. In addition, pay attention to what activities or situations are likely to exacerbate sleepiness. Commonly, sitting or lying down while reading or watching television are likely to induce sleep. This sleepiness might come on during your buffer zone in the hour before your goal bedtime. You may need to do something to counteract it.

Take measures to avoid sleeping outside of your goals.
Any sleep that occurs outside of your goal bedtime and wake time will diminish your desire for sleep at night. If a long period of uninterrupted sleep is a feast, you want to show up hungry, and naps are sleep snacks. If you snack all day, you won't be hungry when the time for feasting arrives. Review your list of activities to stay awake and select the one most likely to be effective for you. Try to select an option that will keep you active, but not something overly stimulating that may interfere with your ability to fall asleep later. If you feel sleepiness coming on, get up and become more active.

Avoid the traps for dozing: times and situations when you are likely to fall asleep. If you can't sit in your comfortable easy chair and watch television

> *Naps are
> sleep snacks.*

without falling asleep, consider sitting in a firm-backed dining room chair instead, or avoid the activity entirely at that time. Enlist the help of others who can wake you if they see you have nodded off. The more you can stay awake during the day, the better you will sleep at night.

Discover ways to enjoy your morning.

If you are not a morning person and have trouble getting out of bed, you may need to really motivate yourself to get up. With sleep deprivation, you may find it very difficult to wake after a short night of sleep. Beyond setting multiple alarms positioned across the room to compel yourself to get out of bed, or having someone else on hand to wake you, you may want to find other means to motivate yourself to rise and shine.

First, reflect on why you might be lingering in bed. What is the problem? If you hate mornings, why is this so? Consider these possible scenarios:

- You may be reluctant to get up because you do not feel particularly well rested. Morning sunlight may help to increase your circadian alerting signal. The fresh air may also help to wake you. If your sleep quality remains poor after adding back sleep time in the next weeks, you might consider conditions that can undermine sleep like sleep apnea.
- You might feel especially warm and comfortable snuggled in bed, avoiding the cool morning air. Perhaps having a comfortable robe at your bedside to throw on before quickly moving to the hot shower would help.

- You may have body pain and wish to continue to rest. Can you keep your morning pain medicine at the bedside to take immediately upon awakening? Is there a way to optimize your pain control by discussing this issue with your doctor?
- Perhaps you have convinced yourself that you will fall asleep again and this is when you get your best sleep. Sleep is often light and fragmented toward morning, as you have already greatly diminished your sleep drive. How successful have you been in the past? Chances are that the results are inconsistent. Extra time in bed may further condition you toward wakefulness and it weakens the drive for sleep the next night.
- You may be avoiding your day, unable to face the anticipated events. You may feel like you have nothing to look forward to. Will lying in bed change this? How could you more productively resolve this issue? Can you give yourself something to look forward to the next day before going to bed?

It can be useful to create a list of ways to motivate yourself to get up at your goal wake time each and every day. Keeping this regular wake time as a fixed anchor, reinforced by morning sunlight exposure, can help to improve your sleep. As you change your morning routine, it will become easier. Review your list of ideas before going to bed and make arrangements to optimize your morning success.

Ways to Help Get Out of Bed in the Morning:
1. Immediately go to the shower to increase alertness.
2. Put on exercise clothes and go to the gym.
3. Take the dog outside.

4.   Feed your pets.

5.   Go for a walk.

6.   Treat yourself to your favorite cup of coffee or tea.

7.   Make a special breakfast.

8.   Visit your favorite local coffee shop.

9.   Arrange a meeting with a friend.

10. Ask someone to call you at a time shortly after your awakening.

11. Schedule an early appointment that you won't want to miss.

12. Assign time for your favorite hobby for first thing in the morning.

13. Reduce the use of sleeping pills that may have morning hangover effects.

14. _____

    _____

15. _____

    _____

16. _____

    _____

17. _____

    _____

18. _____

    _____

19. _____

    _____

20. _____

    _____

How Sleeping Pills Work and the Risks

 Sleeping pills are various medications that are used to remedy insomnia by easing the ability to fall and stay asleep. These over-the-counter and prescription drugs may enhance the depth and amount of sleep obtained. There are dozens of options with different actions, side effects, and costs. How do sleeping pills work? What are the potential short- and long-term side effects? If you are interested in stopping a sleep aid, how should this best be achieved? As sleep improves, this may be the week to begin setting aside these potentially harmful medications.

Before exploring the extensive list of potential sleeping pills, let's take a moment to recognize how commonly these drugs are being used. Without question, the use of medications marketed to improve sleep has exploded over the last decades. These may include unregulated supplements with dubious benefits, over-the-counter "PM" sleep aids, and some of the most widely recognized and prescribed drugs. According to the Centers for Disease Control, between 2005 and 2010, about 4 percent of adults 20 and older had used a sleeping pill in the previous month. IMH Health, an organization that tracks drug data, reported that 59 million sleeping pills were prescribed in 2012, up from 56 million in 2008. Market research also revealed a tripling in sleep aid prescriptions from 1998 to 2006 among young adults aged 18 to 24. Either our collective sleep is rapidly worsening or we are increasingly being sold a solution found in a bottle. These are troubling statistics, especially in light of the potential side effects that shall be discussed later.

Medications that are used to aid sleep fall into two broad

categories based on their potential mechanisms of action: they may enhance signals for sleepiness or block signals for wakefulness (see Figure 11). The balance of specific chemicals in the brain may affect the overall state of consciousness. When levels of the sleep-inducing chemicals increase, sleep onset and persistence is more likely to occur.

The chemical signals that induce sleep include: melatonin, galanin, gamma-aminobutyric acid (GABA), adenosine, and cytokines. Many sleeping pills augment these effects. As you may recall, adenosine levels also increase with prolonged wakefulness and this is the chemical that has been building up with sleep consolidation. Reducing or blocking these chemicals induces wakefulness. On the other side of the balance are the chemical signals that promote wakefulness. These include histamine, orexin/hypocretin, norepinephrine, acetylcholine, serotonin, and dopamine. Many sleeping pills work by blocking these chemicals, such

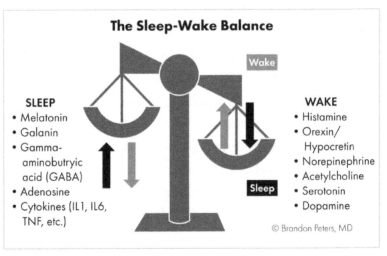

Figure 11

as antihistamines found in the over-the-counter "PM" drugs. If these chemicals are increased—such as occurs with stimulant medications—wakefulness is promoted.

The Major Classes of Sleeping Pills

Substances have been used to enhance sleep for millennia. Prescription drugs sold for these purposes have been around for more than 100 years. These sleep aids can be grouped into over-the-counter options (including supplements sold as pills, liquids, patches, and sprays) and prescription medications. Let's explore some of the medications that exist and how they work.

If you peel away the fancy packaging and marketing, over-the-counter sleep aids contain many of the same basic ingredients. Supplements are not regulated by the U.S. Food and Drug Administration (FDA), so you should use caution, as there is no enforcement in regards to the quality and manufacturing standards. There also may be little scientific evidence demonstrating the drug's effectiveness.

Diphenhydramine

This antihistamine causes sleepiness as a side effect. It is frequently used to treat allergic reactions. It is available as Benadryl and found in most of the "PM" drugs, including Tylenol PM, Advil PM, and Aleve PM. It is also sold as ZzzQuil. Side effects include dryness and urinary retention. There may be morning hangover effects with sleepiness or a drugged feeling upon awakening. It is linked to long-term memory problems (more on this later) and older people may have more side effects.

Doxylamine

Another example of an antihistamine, doxylamine also treats allergies and causes sleepiness or drowsiness as a side effect. It is the active ingredient found in Unisom, NyQuil, and related products. The side effects are similar to diphenhydramine. Unfortunately, it has a higher risk of worsening insomnia and leading to dependence.

Melatonin

Melatonin is a hormone naturally produced by the brain's pineal gland during sleep. It reinforces the circadian rhythm and may modestly improve insomnia as a supplement. Attractive as a more natural option, there is still the potential for side effects. These include nightmares and daytime sleepiness, especially at higher doses.

L-Tryptophan

Often taken as a supplement, it is an amino acid, one of the building blocks of protein. The body creates melatonin (through conversion to serotonin) from tryptophan. It is found in high levels in certain foods, including turkey, soybeans, egg whites, pork chops, and parmesan cheese. Despite the logical possibility that it may enhance sleep, there is minimal evidence supporting its use as a reliable sleep aid.

Serotonin

Similar in structure to tryptophan, serotonin is metabolized into melatonin with the sleep-promoting properties described. There may be risks associated with excessive serotonin use, especially when taking selective serotonin reuptake inhibitor (SSRI) medications for anxiety or depression that increase serotonin levels within the brain.

GABA

Gamma-amino butyric acid (GABA) is the primary neurotransmitter in the brain that slows the activity of neurons. Formed from glutamate, it acts by opening chloride channels and reducing the electrical conduction of cells. Many medications, including prescription benzodiazepine sleeping pills, work by activating receptors for GABA. Similar medications may treat seizures and spasticity.

Valerian Root

Since ancient Greek times, this herb has been used for its sedating properties to aid sleep. Although considered safe, the exact mechanism of how it works remains unknown. It may relieve anxiety. Most research suggests no significant response to the supplement to improve parameters of sleep.

Kava-kava

Found in the Western Pacific, including Hawaii, this plant has been used for its sedative properties and anxiety relief for thousands of years. It may affect receptors for GABA, serotonin, and dopamine. It has not been well studied for its impacts on sleep. Unfortunately, there have been significant safety concerns related to its use. It may cause hepatotoxicity, leading to liver failure. As a consequence, its use has been restricted in Europe. Its use is discouraged due to the potential for these serious risks.

Chamomile

Often consumed as a tea, chamomile is also found in tablets, pow-
ders, and gelcaps used as sleep aids. It may cause sleepiness and
relieve anxiety. Limited scientific research has not demonstrated
a benefit in its use to improve insomnia. There are very few side
effects, but it may cause skin irritation if used topically.

Marijuana

Smoked or ingested, marijuana likely exerts its effects through
the cannabinoid receptors of the central nervous system. There
are over 100 types of cannabinoids found in marijuana, but
delta-9 tetrahydrocannabinol (THC) and cannabidiol (CBD)
occur in the largest amount. It seems that CBD may have a more
positive effect on anxiety relief and sleep, but further research
into potential harms is needed.

When insomnia comes to the attention of a physician, a prescription for a medication to improve sleep inevitably follows. These
drugs can be grouped into a handful of major classes with varying
actions and potential side effects:

Barbiturates

One of the oldest classes of medicine, barbiturates have been used
as anesthesia for surgery and to resolve intractable seizures. In
1912, phenobarbital was first introduced as a hypnotic to treat
insomnia. Due to the extremely high risks of overdose and withdrawal, barbiturates are no longer prescribed as a sleep aid.

Benzodiazepines

Discovered by accident in 1955, benzodiazepine medications relieve anxiety, alcohol withdrawal, seizures, and insomnia. Enhancing the effects of GABA, the drug reduces the activity of neurons by affecting chloride channels. These medications have generic names that end in "-lam" or "-pam." The benzodiazepines include:

- Lorazepam (Ativan)
- Clonazepam (Klonopin)
- Diazepam (Valium)
- Alprazolam (Xanax)
- Estazolam (ProSom)
- Temazepam (Restoril)
- Triazolam (Halcion)

The benzodiazepine medications may have higher rates of associated abuse and increase the risk of falls, delirium, and long-term memory problems. There is the risk for overdose, especially when taken with alcohol. Due to the potential for withdrawal when use is abruptly stopped, these medications must be tapered under the supervision of a physician to ensure side effects (such as seizures) do not occur.

Antidepressants and Antipsychotics

Trazodone, an old antidepressant, is often used at lower doses as a sleep aid. It may increase deeper sleep with few known long-term side effects. Like many sleeping pills, it may only modestly improve sleep. Silenor (doxepin) is another antidepressant that is infrequently used for insomnia. In addition, psychiatrists may prescribe Seroquel (quetiapine), an atypical antipsychotic medication, to alleviate insomnia. This may be used in older people with delirium, though the long-term safety is concerning, as it may be associated with increased mortality.

Benzodiazapine receptor agonists

Many of the most widely prescribed medications for insomnia work as benzodiazepine receptor agonists. They affect GABA by augmenting its chemical receptors in the brain. Developed over the past 30 years, as hypnotics they seem to have significant transient effects on memory, masking the time spent awake at night. The most common medications in this class include:

- Zolpidem (Ambien, Ambien CR, Intermezzo)
- Eszopiclone (Lunesta)
- Zaleplon (Sonata)

Some formulations, such as Intermezzo and Sonata, have a shorter half-life and can be taken in the middle of the night following awakenings. There are considerable risks with these drugs. Their use may be associated with sleep behaviors and impacts on morning driving, especially in women. There may also be increased long-term risks of dementia, falls, and overall mortality.

Melatonin Agonists

A few medications aid sleep by acting on the receptors for melatonin within the brain. Rozerem, sold as the generic ramelteon, seems to be most effective in aiding the quicker onset of sleep.

Hetlioz (or tasimelteon) is used to treat the Non-24 circadian disorder in blind people.

Orexin Antagonist

Finally, a novel medication is available that reduces the orexin signal for wakefulness. Sold as Belsomra (or suvorexant), it seems to have modest benefits on insomnia and improves sleep maintenance. The loss of orexin is frequently associated with narcolepsy and accounts for the excessive daytime sleepiness that occurs with the disorder.

How Effective Are Sleeping Pills Really?

To be honest, it is shocking how relatively inconsequential the benefits of sleeping pills are when put under rigorous scientific research. This is not to belittle their potential current or former benefit to you, but the impacts on the ability to fall asleep, spend less time awake at night, and sleep more are modest at best.

In 2017, the American Academy of Sleep Medicine published a clinical practice guideline for physicians on the use of sleeping pills to treat chronic insomnia. After thorough review of the body of scientific knowledge, there was weak evidence for their recommendations, suggesting inadequate research and clinical uncertainty. It may be most telling to review their summary of what the research tells us about the effectiveness of some of the most widely prescribed drugs compared to the effects of placebo (see Figure 12).

Effects of Sleeping Pills on Sleep Parameters Based on Research

	Average Reduction in Sleep Onset Latency	Average Reduction in Time Spent Awake at Night	Increase in Total Sleep Time
Ambien (zolpidem)	5–12 minutes	25 minutes	29 minutes
Belsomra (suvorexant)	8 minutes	16–28 minutes	10 minutes
Diphenhydramine	8 minutes	--	12 minutes
Lunesta (eszopiclone)	14 minutes	10–14 minutes	28–57 minutes
Melatonin	9 minutes	--	--
Rozerem (ramelteon)	9 minutes	--	--
Sonata (zaleplon)	10 minutes	--	--
Trazodone	10 minutes	8 minutes	--

Figure 12: Adapted from Sateia MJ et al. "Clinical practice guideline for the pharmacologic treatment of chronic insomnia in adults: an American Academy of Sleep Medicine clinical practice guideline. *J Clin Sleep Med.* 2017;13(2):307–349.

There are a few important takeaway messages from this information. First, these prescription drugs have been approved by the FDA as treatments for chronic insomnia based on scientific evidence that suggests, on average, they can help you to fall asleep just 10 minutes faster. Moreover, they help to reduce the time awake in the night by a paltry 10 to 30 minutes. As a result, the total sleep time increases by similar amounts. (Consider how well you have done with the changes from this past week and the impressive impacts of CBT-I on these measures as discussed earlier.) These reductions do not imply that sleep has normalized. Someone could still have insomnia. Moreover, it is unlikely that these modest benefits will even last.

You don't take medications to feel hungry, so why should you need a medication to feel sleepy? The good news is that you don't need medications to feel sleepy either. You can sleep more normally with the behavioral changes introduced in this program and get away from the use of sleeping pills. Short-term use of these medications may have a role, but use beyond 2 weeks is discouraged. National physician groups, including the American College of Physicians in 2016, have shifted to recommending insomnia therapy as the first-line choice of treatment—and for good reason.

> You don't take medications to feel hungry...you don't need medications to feel sleepy either.

The Dark Side of Sleeping Pills

Before using any medication, it is important to fully and completely consider the risks and alternatives. The risks associated with sleep aids may also motivate you to stop using a drug that likely has only modest benefits. All insomnia medications have potential side effects, and some are quite serious.

Many of these pills are hypnotics, meaning that they affect your memory. They make it hard to remember the time that is spent awake, and this can lead to sleep behaviors such as sleepwalking, eating, and driving. Older people are more likely to fall at night and suffer from hip fractures. In 2012, a study in the *British*

Medical Journal showed that people taking sleeping pills were five times as likely to die over 2½ years compared to those who did not. There seems to be an association between heavy use and a higher incidence of cancer. Recent studies also suggest that, across multiple drug classes (antihistamines, benzodiazepines, and others), the long-term use of sleeping pills may lead to an increased risk of memory problems and dementia. Is it worth it?

Beyond these potential risks, those who use sleeping pills gradually become tolerant, requiring higher doses to get the same effects after repeated exposure. It seems that over time the pills just stop working. It is less likely with occasional use. **Tolerance** is partly due to changes that occur within the brain to down-regulate the response to the drug. The speed at which this tolerance develops may also be dependent on frequency of use, dose, age, sex, weight, and the function of the liver or kidneys.

Over time, the chronic use of sleeping pills may lead to physical or psychological **dependence**. You may come to rely on the drug and without it you may psychologically start to feel a little nervous. Overuse, including the use of higher than recommended doses or use in combination with alcohol, may cause overdose and death. Sudden cessation of benzodiazepine medications may also cause physical withdrawal and even seizures. When any of the prescription medications for sleep are abruptly discontinued, there may be rebound insomnia.

Rebound insomnia causes the ability to sleep to worsen. This may last several days, but fortunately these effects fade. If you are taking a medication for insomnia, and you decide to try to stop it, but as soon as you do your sleep dramatically worsens, what would you do? You go right back to taking it, convinced that without it you are unable to sleep. This is a known side effect to the use of sleeping pills and one that drug companies have no motivation to correct. If you give yourself a few days for your sleep to reset, your sleep can normalize. It can be helpful to minimize the frequency of sleeping pill use and reduce the use of these medications gradually.

Finally, sleeping pills should be tapered gradually under the supervision of your prescribing physician. The doses should be reduced over days to weeks. This reduction will be most successful if done in the context of sleep consolidation. If you are taking sleeping pills, this would be an optimal time to begin to reduce the use of these medications with this guidance. Look back to how poorly you were sleeping last week, on these drugs, and you will recognize that you can sleep better without them if you simply follow the recommendations outlined in this program.

Sleep Efficiency and Beginning Sleep Extension

 It is time to do a little math to determine how successful your first week of sleep consolidation was. In particular, it is necessary to determine your current sleep efficiency. This measurement will be used to make changes to your sleep schedule for next week. Let's review how this calculation is done.

Sleep efficiency is the amount of time that you are spending asleep divided by the total amount of time that you are spending in bed. It is a marker of sleep quality. If you were a perfect sleeper, you would have 100 percent sleep efficiency (sleeping the entire time that you were in bed asleep).

In order to make this calculation, review your sleep log from last week. Determine the amount of time you slept each night, and then average it over the week. (Add up the hours of sleep each night and then divide by the total number of nights.) Do this as well for the average amount of time that you were spending in bed. Then plug these numbers into this formula (see Figure 13).

Now that you have determined your sleep efficiency, you can decide how to change your sleep schedule for this upcoming week and begin the process of sleep extension.

- If your sleep efficiency is **higher than 85 percent**, increase your total time in bed by 15 minutes. If you have daytime sleepiness, you likely need more sleep. This change can be done by either going to bed 15 minutes earlier or alternatively setting the alarm 15 minutes later (don't do both).

- If your sleep efficiency is **80 to 85 percent**, stay on your current schedule for one more week. Continued efforts to optimize your sleep may yield additional benefits. It is also possible, if you do not have daytime sleepiness, that you are currently meeting your sleep needs.

Sleep Efficiency = _____ / _____ × 100%

Average Total Amount of Sleep   Average Total Amount of Time Spent in Bed

© Brandon Peters, MD

Figure 13

- If your sleep efficiency is **less than 80 percent**, review how closely you followed the previous goals for the week. If you were adherent to these recommendations, you should decrease your total time in bed by 15 minutes. Do not spend fewer than 6 hours in bed. If you continue to struggle, consider further evaluation by a sleep specialist.

Stay on this new schedule for at least 7 days before making further changes. This reassessment of your sleep efficiency and further sleep extension will occur on a weekly basis until you are adequately meeting your sleep needs with reduced insomnia.

Conclusion

This week we reviewed your first week of sleep consolidation. We identified areas that may require focused attention for the upcoming week. We discovered the importance of conditioning, learning to associate the bed with sleep by consistently observing stimulus control. We considered ways to stay awake and how to enjoy mornings. We discussed in detail the most common sleeping pills, the limits of their efficacy, potential side effects, and the importance of supervision as the drugs are gradually tapered and discontinued. We learned how to calculate sleep efficiency and how to use this information to begin the process of sleep extension. Focus on these weekly goals and return to this text in 1 week with your completed sleep log.

Week 3 Goals:

- Continue keeping a sleep log (p. 141) to track your progress.
- Observe a fixed wake time by getting up at the same time every day with an alarm clock. Set the alarm clock for a goal wake time of _____.
- Do not check the clock at night. Set the alarm and turn or cover it at night to avoid clock checking.
- Get 15 to 30 minutes of morning sunlight upon awakening (or at sunrise).
- Avoid taking naps unless required for safety (and keep them brief if needed).
- New goal bedtime at _____ with lights out immediately. Spend 60 minutes relaxing before bedtime (using list for ideas). If necessary, stay up later until feeling sleepy.
- If awake for more than 15 minutes at night, by your estimate, get up and go to another room and do something relaxing until feeling sleepy and then come back to bed.
- If you are using sleeping pills, discuss and begin to gradually taper these medications with the supervision of your prescribing doctor.

Note: After your first week of sleep extension, return to this text and begin the next book chapter.

Relaxation Techniques and Mindfulness

Reflection: Changing Negative Thoughts
Education: Mindfulness and Relaxation Training
Goal Setting: Relaxation Techniques

Learning Objectives:

- Reflect on how negative thinking may be impacting your ability to fall asleep.
- Discover ways to change negative thoughts through cognitive therapy techniques.
- Learn about the concepts of mindfulness and reflect on how these may apply to sleep.

- Consider the use of scheduled worry time to help reduce anxiety and racing thoughts and improve the management of stress.
- Understand the role of relaxation techniques and review breathing techniques, progressive muscle relaxation, and guided imagery.
- Review your current sleep log, briefly revisit your program goals, and continue the process of sleep extension based on sleep efficiency.

The Impacts of Mood on Sleep

If you have ever had a fight with someone just before going to bed, you are no doubt quite familiar with the impacts of negative feelings on sleep. Rather than easily dozing off, you will lie there awake. You may ruminate about the situation, your reaction, or what you plan to do about it. Let's consider how negative emotions and the associated thinking impact our ability to fall asleep and begin to identify the degree to which it may be contributing to your insomnia.

Let's imagine that it is 40,000 years ago and you are sleeping in a cave environment. Not only would your sleep pattern be more closely linked to the natural patterns of light and darkness, reinforcing your circadian rhythm, but you will also be subject to potential dangers. Waking at night may serve as an evolutionary advantage: you could be more aware of threats that creep close in the night.

If you woke to discover that there were a lion in your cave, how would your body react? You would get an immediate surge of adrenaline (stress hormone) triggered by the sympathetic nervous system. This is the classic "fight or flight" response, meant to preserve an organism from an external threat. There are measurable changes in the body: pupils dilate to increase visual input,

It is not safe to sleep when we feel stressed.

breathing and blood circulation increase, along with spikes in the heart rate and blood pressure. The ability to sleep (mediated by the balancing parasympathetic influence) is instantly abolished. This is helpful for survival: if you easily fell back asleep after seeing a lion, you wouldn't be long for this world. It is not safe to sleep when we feel stressed.

Fortunately, we no longer sleep in caves with the undesirable possibility of lions or predators prowling and attacking us in the night. Nevertheless, the body still responds to perceived threats and stresses in the exact same way. Modern "lions" are the numerous issues that cause us to feel anxious, upset, or distressed on a daily basis. These triggers include everything from minor annoyances (a noisy neighbor), to social problems (a troubled marriage), to professional turmoil (job insecurity), and numerous other possibilities. There is a lot to keep someone up at night!

Our reactions to these issues, especially if they are not satisfactorily addressed during the day, are truly what keep us awake. If there is a sound at night that wakes you that immediately goes away, you might normally fall back asleep easily. However, if the sound is your neighbor coming home late and again raising a racket that disturbs your sleep—the emotional baggage attached to that noise may cause the awakening to trigger a reaction. As

> *Anxiety, frustration, anger—none of these feelings are conducive to sleep.*

curse words fly through your mind, adrenaline floods your system and your ability to fall back asleep is severely compromised. Anxiety, frustration, anger—none of these feelings are conducive to sleep. If present, you will be kept awake until their influence subsides. When they recur frequently, the bed may become associated with wakefulness and distress and condition insomnia to persist. Reducing their impact may require identifying and restructuring the negative thoughts associated with sleep.

Connecting Sleep-Related Thoughts to Emotions

Take a moment to consider how you react to difficulty falling asleep at the beginning of the night or returning to sleep if you wake in the night. What do you think or tell yourself? Is there a strongly negative emotion attached to this occurrence? Although some people may not develop a pattern of negative thoughts and reactions with difficulty sleeping, it commonly occurs in chronic insomnia. The following exercises may help you to identify these negative thoughts that may cause an emotional reaction that worsens insomnia. Take as much time as is necessary to unpack this baggage. If it does not apply to your situation, you may pass through these questions swiftly and move on to the next section.

First, start by listing any insomnia-related thoughts that you have that cause distress or impact your ability to fall asleep. These thoughts are the "self-talk" that usually occur when you cannot get to sleep at night. (Incidentally, these may have been reduced recently as you work through this program.) To get you started, some examples are provided. Circle any that sound familiar to you and then add your own:

1. I won't be able to function tomorrow.
2. I need to take another sleeping pill.
3. What is wrong with me?
4. I have to do something to get back to sleep.
5. I really can't take this any longer.
6. This isn't working.
7. Why does this keep happening to me?
8. I am never going to be able to sleep normally again.
9. _____

    _____
10. _____

    _____
11. _____

    _____
12. _____

    _____
13. _____

    _____
14. _____

    _____

Now that you have identified some of the predominant thoughts that come up at night as you are lying awake, let's try to identify the emotions that may be attached to these thoughts. If you think to yourself, "I will never be able to get to sleep (or back to sleep) tonight," how would that make you **feel**?

_____

_____

_____

Are there **other thoughts or images** that would immediately follow that initial thought? (i.e., concerns about functioning the next day, when to get up, etc.)

_____

_____

_____

What **action** follows the initial thought, the emotional response, and the associated thoughts that commonly occur? (i.e., take a sleeping pill, turn off the alarm, get up)

_____

_____

_____

Consider some of the other examples of sleep-related thoughts that you listed above. Work through these thoughts in a similar way, identifying the emotional reaction, associated thoughts, and actions that have occurred in the setting of insomnia. After reviewing these patterns, it becomes possible to identify false beliefs and begin to restructure this thinking to aid sleep. Substituting more evidence-based thoughts when these negative thoughts recur can shut down their recurrence.

False Beliefs Interfere with Normal Sleep

The mind is not rational in a state of sleep deprivation. Logic suffers in the emotional swings of fitful sleep. Flights of fancy driven by anxiety may lead to conclusions that seem far-fetched by the light of day. False beliefs are common in insomnia, and testing them by pushing them to their limits can help their recurrence to fade.

Consider the following examples of statements that you may have thought, and may still believe, that may not actually be true. With each idea, note evidence-based commentary that might help to diminish their potential impact:

When I have trouble sleeping, I should try harder.

The more you try to sleep, the less you are actually able to fall asleep. Effort undermines the ability to sleep. When focus is placed on falling asleep, sleep does not occur. The harder you try, the more difficult it becomes. Instead, the mental focus has to be shifted elsewhere for sleep to come.

I should sleep at least 8 hours every night.

Although this number reflects the average sleep needs for a population, this may not reflect your individual sleep need. You may have shorter or longer sleep needs based on your genetics. In addition, the amount of sleep needed changes with aging, with older adults often needing only 7 to 8 hours of sleep to feel rested. When fewer hours of sleep are obtained, sleep quality actually improves. If you spend too much time in bed, exceeding your sleep needs, insomnia worsens as sleep lightens and thins out.

If I don't get enough sleep, I won't be able to function at all tomorrow.

Consider the nights when you have slept especially poorly. The next day, you no doubt felt like you were running on fumes, but it is likely that you were still able to do most (if not all) of the things you were required to do. Chances are that you went to work, took care of the family, completed chores, and accomplished much of what needed to be done. You may not have performed at your best, but you did not have zero function.

Bad nights of sleep occur more often when the prior night was bad.

Consider the patterns of sleep documented in your own sleep logs over the past weeks, especially the baseline sleep log that you completed. How do bad nights of sleep relate to good nights? Is there any regular pattern that you recognize? Contrary to this belief, you may note that a short night of sleep will build the sleep drive and this increased desire for sleep can improve sleep on a subsequent night. It is common to have one or two bad nights of sleep followed by an especially good night. This sleep drive may be diminished by spending too much time in bed or trying to sleep too much, such as occurs when waking late, taking a nap, or going to bed too early. A shorter night of sleep improves sleep through sleep consolidation. Therefore, a bad night of sleep may actually help you to sleep better if you use the resulting sleep deprivation to your advantage.

I should try to catch up on lost sleep by going to bed early.

If you feel sleep deprived, the best thing to do is to harness this to improve the next night of sleep. Build the sleep drive to be especially strong by staying up later so that you fall asleep faster and, if waking at night, fall back asleep more easily. Keep to a regular bedtime and wake time to reinforce the timing of sleep. It is counterintuitive to stay up later when you have trouble getting enough sleep, but it works to improve sleep quality. Going to bed too early or staying in bed too late in the morning extends the time in bed and worsens insomnia.

Changing Thoughts with Cognitive Therapy

Now that you have identified some of the negative thoughts and false beliefs that might undermine your relationship with sleep, it is possible to begin to challenge these thoughts. The *cognitive* component of cognitive behavioral therapy for insomnia (CBT-I) refers to thoughts, the internal processing that occurs in the setting of difficulty sleeping. As discussed, when these thoughts are linked with negative emotions (especially anxiety), sleep becomes very difficult. If this is bothersome, it can be useful to restructure these thoughts via a rational analysis.

Learning is reinforced through repetition. In a sense, you can learn to have the same thoughts, feelings, and behaviors associated with insomnia. Every time that you get into bed, spend 30 minutes lying awake, begin to worry about how this will impact the next day, try harder to get to sleep, and toss and turn, the pattern is reinforced. You are unwittingly practicing insomnia.

Observing stimulus control (getting up when you aren't sleeping) can help, and so can undermining the thoughts that drive insomnia.

No matter what train of thought interferes with your ability to fall asleep, it is possible to derail it, or at least direct it to a different destination. Sometimes a few challenging questions can be helpful: Is that really true? Do the concerns I have about what could happen correspond to what actually happens? How is this negative thinking helpful to me? What is the evidence for and against this belief? By identifying common thoughts that occur at night, and assessing the evidence during the day, alternative thoughts can be created that may redirect this thinking.

Consider some of the most common thoughts that occur to you at night that may interfere with your ability to get to sleep. What is the situation where this thought is likely to occur? Try to state the thought in a simple sentence. What is the mood associated with the thought (anxiety, depression, anger, frustration, hopelessness, etc.)? In addition to identifying the emotion linked to the thought, try to rate the intensity of the mood by giving it a percentage from 0 to 100 percent. On this scale, 100 percent would represent the instance when you felt that emotion at its greatest intensity *in your entire life*. Now, start to analyze the evidence for and against the idea that you have. Imagine you are a lawyer arguing a case and you want to identify as many pros for, and cons against, the thought as possible. Try to base this on factual evidence of things that actually occur, not beliefs or concerns about what *may* occur. Finally, consider a way to rephrase the thought in a more logical way that better reflects the evidence for the idea. If possible, try to make it more positive. Finally, reassess your mood as you consider this new alternative thought compared to your baseline mood. Use the table on this page to do the analysis.

Complete the table for some of the most common disruptive thoughts that interfere with your sleep at night. Do this as much as is necessary to defuse negative thinking related to your sleep. If the thought comes up, recall that you reviewed the evidence and remind yourself of the alternative thought. This can help to reframe a recurrent experience and lead you down a path that leads to falling asleep easier.

Situation	**Ex.:** In bed
Thought	"If I can't sleep, I won't be able to go to work tomorrow."
Mood (%)	Anxious 80%
Pros (True)	My work performance may not be optimal.
Cons (False)	• I never miss work. • No one notices impairment. • I do good work. • I will get through it.
Alternate Thought	"I may not function optimally, but I will still go to work and do what I need to do."
New Mood (%)	Less anxious 40%

Situation	
Thought	
Mood (%)	
Pros (True)	
Cons (False)	
Alternate Thought	
New Mood (%)	

The Application of Mindfulness to Sleep

 Mindfulness is a practice by which one develops an increased awareness of the present moment, fully sensing the elements of an experience. It is a technique to acknowledge and accept feelings, thoughts, and bodily sensations as they occur. Often incorporated into meditation, yoga, and Buddhist practices, mindfulness can also be helpfully integrated into insomnia therapy to improve sleep by changing our relationship to it.

Consider how these concepts of mindfulness, elucidated in the context of insomnia by psychologists Rachel Manber, PhD, and Alison Siebern, PhD, at Stanford University, may relate to our sleep:

- **Beginner's Mind**: Each night is a brand new chance to have a good night of sleep. Approach it as a blank slate, open to the possibility that something different can occur. Remember that what you had been doing previously was not working, and that changes may lead to the gradual improvement in your sleep that you seek.

- **Non-striving**: This is a lesson you have already learned: you can't force sleep to happen. The more you focus on falling asleep, the less you are able to get to sleep. Sleep should be allowed to occur naturally, when you have a strong sense of sleepiness. Effort undermines sleep and becomes counterproductive.

- **Letting Go**: Sometimes we worry about the consequences of a poor night of sleep and how it will impact us the next day. Stress may interfere with falling asleep. We become anxious, frustrated, or upset. None of these feelings are conducive to sleep. Rather than increasing pressure to sleep perfectly, let go and allow sleep to occur.

- **Non-judging**: Remember that it is normal to wake up at night: to roll over, adjust the covers, respond to noise, or go to the bathroom. If after waking, someone changes position and goes right back to sleep, this is not a bother. It is only a negative reaction to the awakening that may cause it to become more prolonged. Judging waking as abnormal undermines an easy transition back to sleep.

- **Acceptance**: There may be times that you get into bed, or wake at night, and simply can't get to sleep. Accept this. Get up, do something relaxing, and return to bed when you are feeling more sleepy. This will help to recondition the bed as a place for sleep. It will strengthen your sleep drive. It will help you to sleep better. If you are struggling one night, no matter the reason, get up and reset your sleep.

- **Trust**: Trust that you can sleep normally. Your sleep system—the sleep drive and circadian rhythm—will always help you to sleep better. This system cannot be broken. It will help to compensate for shorter periods of sleep by providing deeper, less fragmented recovery sleep. You can always use these abilities to help yourself to sleep better. Sleep deprivation will always increase your desire for sleep, and properly timed light exposure (usually in the morning) can help keep you on schedule.

- **Patience**: These changes take time. This program is designed to last 6 weeks because it usually takes about 6 weeks to effectively make these adjustments. If you have had insomnia for months or even years, give yourself the time you need to gradually change these behaviors and habits. In a relatively short period of time, you will make gains to improve both the quality and quantity of your sleep. Moreover, you will learn a set of skills that will help you to sleep better the rest of your life.

Reflect on your own sleep experiences and how these may have started to change as part of this therapy program. Be confident that you can continue to make adjustments to optimize your sleep over the coming weeks.

Managing Stress with a List and Scheduled Worry Time

Sleep is often worsened during periods of stress. These triggers might be transient or persistent. If the situation resolves, we might be able to return to normal sleep fairly quickly. Unfortunately, sometimes this stress is chronic and we must find new ways to manage our responses to it. It can sometimes be helpful to schedule a "worry time" each day to assess and work through stress that may undermine the ability to sleep.

It is best to find a time in the late afternoon or early evening to take stock of the day. Don't do it right before bedtime. Protect this time, returning to it each day. As you get started, it can be helpful to create a comprehensive written list of stressors. This might be accomplished by keeping an ongoing worry journal or by updating a list kept on a piece of paper, a document on a computer, a memo note on a phone, or in an email sent to yourself. It is private—not meant to be shared with anyone else.

List all the sources of stress in your life. These are situations or thoughts that lead to stress, worry, tension, concern, pressure, and anxiety—whatever words you want to use. Reflect on the various stresses that occur in life. These might be related to professional, financial, relationship, family, or health issues. Whatever the nature of the concern, write it down. In a sense, this is naming evil, putting words to something that might be weighing you down. The first day it takes some time to create the list, but you can simply update it on subsequent days: our stressors don't change much from day to day.

It is not enough to simply stew on these sources of stress. In the second column of your list, brainstorm ideas for ways that you might begin to address some of these problems. What is the plan to resolve the situation? What might you do to help alleviate the source of stress? Let's take an example and suppose that your source of stress is the fact that you forgot to do your taxes this year. You write the word "Taxes" in the first column. In thinking of a plan to address this source of stress, you begin to write ideas: "Gather the necessary tax documents," "Schedule a visit with the accountant," "Submit the required paperwork," and "Pay the back taxes and penalties." You have very specific tasks to accomplish that will help to address the source of stress. As you revisit the list each day, you cross off the things that you have done. Over time, as the action items are achieved, you also can entirely cross off a source of stress. You may tackle the easier issues, picking the low-hanging fruit on the list, but you are still gradually working to reduce stress in your life.

Consider the use of the template on the following page to create your own worry list, dividing the page into the two columns as suggested.

Certainly some items listed may cause significant stress and may have little (or no) chance of favorable resolution. Perhaps you have written down that you are stressed because your loved one has been diagnosed with terminal cancer. Though you cannot fix this problem, you can still identify helpful things to do. Perhaps you would find it beneficial to read more about the condition, go to the next doctor's appointment to be supportive, send flowers with a thoughtful card, arrange a long visit to reminisce about better times, or lend comfort in other ways. These interventions may not resolve the cancer, but they may still be of help.

There may be some things on your list that you don't have a plan to resolve. At least for now, there is nothing to do about it. This is helpful as well: to acknowledge that something is out of your hands, and, for today, you have to let it go. Perhaps things will change by tomorrow and you will come up with a new plan, but for today you simply put it on your list and *let it go*.

Scheduled worry time can almost become a pressure relief valve. By writing these things down, you don't have to constantly remind yourself of what causes you stress. If you think of something at an inopportune time (such as when you wake at night with your mind racing), remind yourself that it is on your list. You will return to it tomorrow during your scheduled worry time. For now, it's time to get back to sleep. (It can even be helpful to have a piece of paper and pen at your bedside to write down new things that may come to mind.) As often as the worried thought recurs outside of worry time, you redirect to this same conclusion: "I will come back to it tomorrow."

Scheduled worry time helps to identify, organize, and prioritize these concerns. By reflecting on and working through an action plan, you can begin to make changes that will help you to move forward. As you revisit the list each day, you get a sense of accomplishment as you begin to complete the actionable items and resolve stress. Other sources of stress may gradually fade away. It also provides an opportunity to defer anxious thoughts that may not currently have an obvious resolution.

List of Worries	Solutions or Ways to Address

Creating a List of Ways to Cope with Stress

Beyond a scheduled time to manage a list of worries, it may also be a worthwhile endeavor to identify ways that in the past you have found helpful to cope with stress. Create a list of activities, hobbies, and pastimes that you find effectively reduce stress for you. This list will be individualized to your own preferences, but some suggestions are provided to get you started. It is possible that someone may find a particular activity stressful that someone else finds relaxing, so make it personal.

If you are feeling particular stressed, during the day or at night, revisit this list of ideas to select something to do to help reduce your anxiety. When it is difficult to shut down the mind at night due to racing thoughts, it might be especially important to spend the hour before the goal bedtime engaged in relaxing activities. The other relaxation techniques described later in the next section may also be helpful. If you find that your anxiety persists, or seems overwhelming and no longer manageable, you may consider getting additional evaluation and treatment by your doctor (as discussed in the next chapter).

Ways of Coping with Stress

1. Go for a long walk.
2. Watch your favorite movie or TV show.
3. Read a book.
4. Arrange a coffee date with your best friend to talk.
5. Exercise.
6. Journal about your concerns.
7. Spend time with your family or friends.
8. Plan and take a vacation.

9. Do some breathing exercises.

10. _____

_____

11. _____

_____

12. _____

_____

13. _____

_____

14. _____

_____

15. _____

_____

Using Relaxation Techniques to Fall Asleep Faster

 There are many different methods for relaxing. Fortunately, there is no right or wrong approach. Your goal should be to relax both your mind and your body. Consider using the associated audio file found with the online program to practice the suggested breathing, progressive muscle relaxation, and guided imagery described below. Once you have mastered the patterns, you will likely be able to do it without either a written or audio guide.

These techniques can be especially helpful as a means to distract yourself to fall asleep. Rather than creating effort to fall asleep, or worrying about what might happen if you don't fall asleep, focus the mind on these various relaxation techniques.

This cognitive distraction can be used at the beginning of the night, right after you crawl into bed, or after an awakening in the night. You will discover that giving the mind a focus will help you to fall asleep faster. You are not trying to fall asleep, you are in bed and feeling sleepy, and after a few minutes of distraction, you fall asleep.

If you get all the way through the techniques—which often takes about 15 minutes—this might be a cue to get up and come back to bed later when you are feeling more sleepy. This can help to reinforce adherence to stimulus control, which aids the conditioning to associate the bed with sleep. As with any skill, the more you practice, the easier it will become. The following exercises are recommended to be used to aid relaxation:

Breathing

1. Find a quiet environment where you will not be interrupted or distracted.
2. Make yourself comfortable and sit or lie in a position that fully supports your body.
3. Remember that your goal is to relax, not to fall asleep.
4. Start by focusing your mind on your breathing. Take deep, slow breaths through your nose, inhaling and exhaling completely.
5. Focus your mind on the tip of your nose, paying attention to the air temperature difference (cold air in, warm air out) and then the movement of the air. Gradually shift your focus to the upper part of your nose, your throat and tongue, and ultimately to your lungs, noting these same differences.

6. Then, imagine filling your lungs in thirds, pausing between each third. Exhale completely and start again, giving yourself a new chance, and try to make the thirds equal.

Muscle Relaxation

1. Start by paying attention to the signals your body is giving you.

2. In turn, you will focus your mind on different parts of your body, both left and right sides. Each area should be tightened, fully tensing up the muscles. This can be held for 5 seconds, 3 seconds, and then 1–2 seconds. After each tightening, completely relax and let all of that tension go.

3. Muscle groups to tighten and relax:

    (1) Toes: scrunch up your toes

    (2) Lower legs: move your foot up at the ankle and tighten the muscles in the lower leg

    (3) Hands: ball up your fists like you are trying to crush a walnut

    (4) Upper arms: show off your biceps

    (5) Shoulders: shrug your shoulders towards your head

    (6) Face: close your eyes tightly, raise your eyebrows with eyes closed, wrinkle up your nose, and grimace or smile in an exaggerated way

Guided Imagery

Imagine a place you have been that you found very relaxing and calming, a place where you were completely at peace. Consider a favored vacation spot or a place in nature: the beach, a hike in the woods, standing in a meadow or next to a stream. Try to re-create the sensory experience by imagining what you saw, heard, smelled, and felt. Allow yourself to be completely immersed in this relaxing and safe place.

Alternatively, consider other ways to distract yourself. Try to remember the details of a recent dream. Dreams are often quickly forgotten and by trying to bring back the details, you will distract yourself and fall asleep more easily. Imagine winning the lottery and spending the money in fun ways. Start with 300 and slowly count backwards by 6, continually subtracting 6 as you work your way down to zero.

No matter the relaxation technique that you choose, the purpose is to engage your mind in distraction, shift the focus from any effort related to sleep, and let yourself relax completely. These techniques can be effectively used during the day if you are feeling particularly stressed, once you crawl into bed at the start of the night and turn the lights out, or if you wake up during the night and need to get back to sleep.

Continuing Sleep Extension to Meet Program Goals

Take a moment to revisit the goals that you established for the program during the first week. By reviewing your most recent sleep log, you may note improvements in the average time that it is taking to fall asleep or the total time that you are spending awake at night. It is possible that you are consistently meeting your goal wake time and getting morning sunlight. Hopefully you are avoiding daytime naps. Sleepiness may be improving, especially compared to the first week of sleep consolidation, but it may not be resolved. It is also very likely that you still need more sleep and would ultimately like to continue to move your bedtime earlier. It is helpful to acknowledge the gains that you have made in a few short weeks while recognizing where further adjustments are needed to meet your ultimate goals.

As was done last week, use the instructions previously provided to calculate your current sleep efficiency. Moreover, determine if further sleep extension is necessary this week. If appropriate, continue to adjust either your wake time or bedtime incrementally. If you are waking up at your goal, but need more sleep based on the sleep efficiency calculation, go to bed 15 minutes earlier this week. These adjustments will continue over the next weeks until you have met your sleep needs and are feeling fully rested during the day. As this time is added back, you will notice that you are feeling better without a recurrence of insomnia.

Conclusion

This week we have reflected on how negative thinking and the associated emotions may undermine our ability to fall asleep. Through cognitive therapy, we have discovered ways to change these negative thoughts by examining them with a more rational analysis. We have learned about how the concepts of mindfulness can be applied to sleep. We have reviewed the use of scheduled worry time and the creation of a list of ways to improve stress to reduce anxiety that may interfere with sleep. We have practiced relaxation techniques—including breathing, muscle relaxation, and guided imagery—as a way to distract the mind at night to more easily transition to sleep. Finally, we have revisited our program goals to continue the work of sleep extension based on sleep efficiency to fully meet our sleep needs.

Week 4 Goals:

- Continue keeping a sleep log (p. 141) to track your progress.
- Observe a fixed wake time by getting up at the same time every day with an alarm clock. Set the alarm clock for a goal wake time of _____.
- Do not check the clock at night. Set the alarm and turn or cover it at night to avoid clock checking.
- Get 15 to 30 minutes of morning sunlight upon awakening (or at sunrise).
- Avoid taking naps unless required for safety (and keep them brief if needed).
- New goal bedtime at _____ with lights out immediately. Spend 60 minutes relaxing before bedtime (using list for ideas). If necessary, stay up later until feeling sleepy.
- If awake for more than 15 minutes at night, by your estimate, get up and go to another room and do something relaxing until feeling sleepy and then come back to bed.

- Use cognitive therapy, scheduled worry time, and relaxation techniques as needed.
- If you are using sleeping pills, continue to taper or discontinue these medications with the supervision of your prescribing doctor.

Note: After your second week of sleep extension, return to this text and begin the next book chapter.

Coexisting Disorders and Health Impacts

Reflection: Strengths and Weaknesses
Education: Coexisting Disorders
Goal Setting: Tidying Up

Learning Objectives:

- Assess the strengths and weaknesses of your adherence to the treatment recommendations from this past week.
- Reflect on the causes of fatigue that extend beyond sleep.
- Learn about the role of various disorders in exacerbating insomnia, including: obstructive sleep apnea, restless legs syndrome, anxiety, depression, and chronic pain.
- Discover the wide-ranging health impacts of poor sleep and the consequences of sleep deprivation.

- Review basic advice to improve sleep hygiene to identify any factors that may be impacting your sleep.
- Consider if you need to seek further help from a sleep specialist.
- Review your current sleep log, briefly revisit your program goals, and continue the process of sleep extension based on sleep efficiency.

Strengths and Weaknesses of Program Adherence

Congratulations! You have made it to the final phase of the *Sleep Through Insomnia* program. Over the next few weeks, we will work to identify additional areas for improvement, ensure complete resolution of contributions to insomnia, and present a plan to follow for lasting change. The end is in sight: you have already learned much of what you need to know. If you have continued to struggle with insomnia, this chapter will also provide suggestions and a way forward.

Let's take a moment to again reflect on how well you were able to follow the program's recommendations over this past week. Review your sleep log carefully. Consider each of these important goals and assess how well you have been able to adhere to the guidelines. Give each a rating by checking the corresponding box and honestly reflect on your strengths and weaknesses using the following table:

Level of Adherence to Treatment Goals					
(1 = None, 5 = Best)	1	2	3	4	5
Keep a sleep log.	☐	☐	☐	☐	☐
Wake up at the same time every day (even on weekends) by using an alarm clock.	☐	☐	☐	☐	☐
Get out of bed immediately upon awakening.	☐	☐	☐	☐	☐
Get 15–30 minutes of morning sunlight exposure upon awakening (or at sunrise).	☐	☐	☐	☐	☐
Avoid taking naps.	☐	☐	☐	☐	☐
Spend 60 minutes relaxing before bedtime.	☐	☐	☐	☐	☐
Go to bed when feeling sleepy and turn out the lights immediately.	☐	☐	☐	☐	☐
If awake for more than 15 minutes at night, by your estimate, get up and go to another room and do something relaxing until feeling sleepy and then come back to bed.	☐	☐	☐	☐	☐
Do not check the clock at night.	☐	☐	☐	☐	☐
As needed, use relaxation techniques to reduce anxiety.	☐	☐	☐	☐	☐
Taper or discontinue the use of sleeping pills.	☐	☐	☐	☐	☐
Other personal goal:	☐	☐	☐	☐	☐

How have you been doing? Continue to reinforce how closely you follow these recommendations. If you have identified areas of weakness, do your best to improve this week. Consider additional ways that you might be successful. Enlist the help of others to keep you on track toward reaching your goals. Careful adherence will maximize your success in the next week—and in the months and years beyond, after completion of the program.

Causes of Fatigue and Reasons for Feeling Tired

As discussed earlier, sleepiness and fatigue differ in important ways. Sleepiness is the strong desire for sleep that immediately precedes falling asleep. Feeling sleepy or drowsy may be enhanced through sleep consolidation and ease the transition to sleep and resolve insomnia. Sleep that is of sufficient quantity and quality will be restorative, diminishing these levels of sleepiness. In contrast, fatigue or tiredness may not correspond to the ability to fall asleep.

Fatigue, tiredness, exhaustion, low energy, feeling generally unwell—these are distinct feelings from sleepiness, with unique causes and solutions. One can feel extremely physically fatigued to the point of exhaustion after physical exertion like running a marathon. Muscles may begin to fail. There may be heaviness in the limbs. The body may even be stressed to the point that organ systems are strained and begin failing. Yet, even in this state of perilous fatigue, one may not necessarily feel sleepy or have a desire or ability to fall asleep. The same is true in the context of insomnia: other causes may need to be sought if fatigue persists and undermines daytime function, even as sleep improves.

Some of the reasons for feeling tired may have nothing to do with your sleep. Diet, exercise, infections, medical conditions, and even medications may play a role. It may be necessary to consider the impact of these issues on your well-being. Review the following list and identify any factors that may have an impact on you and your health:

Diet

The intake of certain foods may lead to lethargy, bloating, and feeling tired during the day, especially after lunch. Keep a food journal to identify any potential foods that worsen how you feel after eating. Increase intake of lean protein, grains, and vegetables. Consider these contributions:

- Heavy foods (often fried, calorie-dense foods high in fat content)
- Processed and fast foods (high in sugar, salt, and preservatives)
- Foods with high melatonin and tryptophan content (for example, tart cherries and turkey, respectively)
- Alcohol
- Gluten-rich foods in the setting of sensitivity and celiac disease
- Other sensitivities or food allergies
- Hydration (ensure you are drinking enough water)
- Caffeine (as it wears off, it may cause a "crash" in energy levels, often 4 to 6 hours later)

Exercise

Normal levels of physical activity and regular exercise enhance sleep. Evaluate whether you are getting the right amount of activity to keep you energized. Find the right balance between doing too little—or doing too much. Participate in activities that you enjoy, aiming to get 30 to 60 minutes of exercise daily. Walking, bicycling, and swimming are encouraged. Maintain a healthy body weight.

Infections

Often associated with other signs or symptoms (including fever), unrecognized infections may contribute to fatigue. Urinary tract infections (UTIs) more commonly affect women. Yeast infections, especially with *Candida albicans*, may occur. Sinus infections or pneumonia may affect the respiratory system, leading to congestion and cough. Consider routine evaluation by your doctor for appropriate testing, if suspected.

Medical Problems

Due to the strain placed on the body, many medical conditions contribute to feelings of fatigue. Some of the most common include:

- Hypothyroidism
- Anemia (possibly associated with low blood-iron levels)
- Constipation
- Chronic pain
- More serious conditions (cancer, multiple sclerosis, Parkinson's disease, etc.)

Medications

Prescription, over-the-counter, and supplemental medications may have effects (or side effects) that contribute to fatigue. Review your medication list with your health care provider or pharmacist to identify any that may have a role and discuss the risks and benefits before discontinuing any prescribed therapy. In particular, be aware of sleeping pills that may have long half-lives and morning hangover effects. If possible, correlate the timing of initiation or increase in dose of any medications and the worsening of fatigue. Common agents to consider include:

- Antidepressants
- Pain medications
- Other medications that act on the central nervous system (brain)
- Beta-blockers for cardiac conditions and high blood pressure (atenolol, carvedilol, metoprolol, propranolol, etc.)
- Antihistamines (diphenhydramine, doxylamine)
- Supplements containing serotonin, tryptophan, melatonin, or valerian root

Other Causes

Beyond these issues, and others to be reviewed in a moment, consider a few additional reasons for feeling tired. Don't forget about the role of the natural dip in the circadian rhythm that occurs in mid-afternoon. Boredom may lead to poor energy levels. You may feel like you have nothing better to do than to sleep. A restricted lifestyle, with prolonged periods of rest or lying down, may cause physical discomfort. Try to maintain normal activities, including household chores, running errands, and socializing. Eye fatigue due to prolonged near focus (such as with screens) causing blurred vision and twitching eyelids may also have a role.

If you have identified potential causes of fatigue, tiredness, or exhaustion that may be impacting you, consider the need for further evaluation or management of these issues. Make some simple lifestyle changes to see if you feel better. As needed, seek further treatment. Also keep these factors in mind as we review the role of other coexisting sleep, mood, and pain disorders that may occur in chronic insomnia and often cause it to persist if left unaddressed.

What If It Is Not Just Insomnia?

From the start of this program (recall: "Know thyself."), there has been an emphasis on considering other potential contributors to chronic insomnia. This is not by mistake. Insomnia rarely occurs in isolation. It is often the product of other conditions that perpetuate difficulty sleeping. Over the past weeks, efforts have been made to remedy most of the potential cognitive and behavioral issues that reinforce insomnia. Especially if you continue to wake frequently at night, or have struggled to realize the benefits of the program, pay close attention. Insomnia may frequently coexist with various disorders that affect sleep, mood, and pain. Improvements may be limited if the underlying cause persists.

Now we begin the final push to clear away factors that may undermine the best intentions and efforts. Let's revisit the potential role of a handful of medical and psychiatric conditions that may play a role in persistent insomnia:

Obstructive Sleep Apnea

The strength of the evidence for a relationship between untreated obstructive sleep apnea and resulting insomnia cannot be overstated. From founders of the field of sleep medicine, including Christian Guilleminault, MD, and William Dement, MD, PhD, at Stanford University, the link has been highlighted since 1973 when "Insomnia with sleep apnea: a new syndrome" was published in the journal *Science*. They described the phenomenon by which disturbances in breathing trigger arousals (brief awakenings) that cause a transition from deep to light sleep or to full wakefulness. Those who suffer from it may complain of insomnia, not recognizing that frequently sleep apnea may be what wakes you—and insomnia is what keeps you awake. Insomnia may improve some with therapy, but the awakenings may persist if the sleep apnea is left untreated. Sleeping pills may also seem to fail in the setting of the sleep-related breathing disorder. Each abnormal breathing event is associated with a burst of cortisol, or stress hormone, as oxygen levels drop and an awakening is necessary to restore normal breathing.

Even mild sleep apnea may not be so mild. It may consist of awakenings that occur up to 15 times *per hour* of sleep! The sleep is fragmented and its quality is greatly undermined. Imagine someone poking you in the ribs every 4 minutes all night long. Even 8 hours of sleep like that wouldn't feel restful, and that fragmentation is exactly what happens with sleep apnea. This condition is worsened during REM sleep when the muscles of the body are relaxed so that dream-enactment does not occur. REM sleep occurs at 2-hour intervals and is concentrated toward morning. These early-morning awakenings may make it hard to fall back asleep, as the drive for sleep has been greatly diminished. Women are more likely to experience insomnia as a symptom of sleep apnea, especially after menopause.

The incidence of sleep apnea among patients who present to sleep clinics for insomnia complaints is extremely high. As reported at the American Academy of Sleep Medicine meeting in 2017, the high incidence of coexisting sleep apnea may be overlooked and undermine the efficacy of insomnia therapy. In a group of 199 people (63 percent women and an average age of 60.7 years) enrolled in insomnia therapy with me, 74 percent had sleep apnea based on testing. Only 10 percent of the population had a negative sleep study. The remaining 16 percent went untested, despite suspicions in some of underlying sleep apnea contributing to their complaints (see Figure 14). Interestingly, those who failed therapy—with stable sleep efficiency despite efforts to adhere to treatment—had a higher incidence of sleep apnea at 80 percent.

Unfortunately, many people with insomnia are treated with sleeping pills that do nothing to address the underlying cause. Chronically, if sleep apnea remains untreated, the repeated drops in blood oxygen levels may stress and decimate cell populations in the brain that need a lot of oxygen, namely the hippocampus that is responsible for memory formation. As a result, untreated sleep apnea is associated with the development of dementia. Those who are placed on sleeping pills may face a similar fate, perhaps due to the unrecognized sleep apnea that goes on for decades.

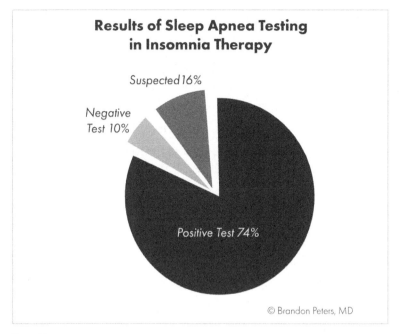

Results of Sleep Apnea Testing in Insomnia Therapy

Suspected 16%

Negative Test 10%

Positive Test 74%

© Brandon Peters, MD

Figure 14

If you are struggling with insomnia therapy, if you can't stay asleep and keep waking in the night, if you have early morning awakenings, if your sleep efficiency is stubbornly not improving, if you aren't where you want to be in the program, and if you experienced intolerable daytime sleepiness, mood changes, or increased pain with sleep consolidation—think about sleep apnea. Get tested. Get treated.

Restless Legs Syndrome

As discussed previously, restless legs symptoms may interfere with your ability to get to sleep. Often experienced when lying down at night, restless legs syndrome is characterized by an uncomfortable feeling associated with a psychiatric urge to move that is relieved by movement. Though most often felt in the legs, any body part may be involved. When severe, the disturbance to sleep onset may be profound. It affects about 10 percent of people and may be associated with iron deficiency and other medical conditions. Medications may be effective, including dopamine agonists (such as pramipexole and ropinirole) as well as other options. If left untreated, insomnia may persist.

Narcolepsy

Among the various sleep disorders, narcolepsy is relatively uncommon, but it still affects nearly 1 in 2,000 people. Caused by the destruction of hypocretin- or orexin-containing cells within the hypothalamus of the brain, this disease leads to lifelong consequences. Beyond fragmented sleep and insomnia complaints, excessive daytime sleepiness, sleep paralysis, sleep-associated hallucinations, and cataplexy (weakness associated with emotions) may occur. Medications may provide relief of these symptoms, but unfortunately there is no cure.

Anxiety

Sleep and mood walk hand in hand. If you don't sleep well, mood worsens. After a bad night of sleep, you may be cranky, short-tempered, grouchy, tense, and irritable. After a great night of sleep, mood lifts and others may notice your improved demeanor. This is due to the effects of sleep on the frontal lobe of the brain, an area

> *Anxiety is an accelerant for the fire of insomnia.*

responsible for executive functions such as higher-level thinking, reasoning, problem-solving, planning, and organization
as well as sociability (i.e., getting along with others). Untreated
mood disorders like anxiety and depression can also negatively
affect sleep, thus creating a bidirectional relationship. Anxiety
is an accelerant for the fire of insomnia. Managing anxiety may
help to ease the ability to both fall and stay asleep, especially if
sleep itself is a source of anxious thoughts. Medications, relaxation techniques, and other therapy may be helpful. Consultation
with a health care provider, including the involvement of a psychologist or psychiatrist, may be needed to fully resolve this
coexisting disorder.

Depression

Beyond feeling down, depression denotes
a state of profound mood impairment
with sadness and a loss of interest that
affects daily function and may be associated with changes in sleep, energy,
concentration, and appetite. It may be
associated with feelings of guilt, a lack

*Sleep and
mood walk
hand in hand.*

of interest (called apathy), and restricted activities. Insomnia is a
known risk factor for depression, increasing the likelihood of its
occurrence by 4 to 40 times (depending on the population studied). Both are linked to a higher risk of suicide, and anyone with
suicidal thoughts is encouraged to reach out to the National Suicide
Prevention Lifeline by calling toll-free 1-800-273-8255. As above,
medications and other therapy may be helpful, and consultation
with a health care provider is recommended.

Chronic Pain

Sleep seems to have a critical role in reducing the experience of pain during wakefulness, and untreated pain can make it hard to fall asleep. Research suggests that slow-wave sleep, predominant in the first hours of the night, may be especially important to repair the body's tissues. Sleep deprivation, or sleep of poor quality, worsens pain tolerance. Fibromyalgia, a chronic pain condition that typifies this relationship, may be improved when associated sleep disorders (like sleep apnea) are treated and sleep quality is optimized. No matter the cause, effective treatment of pain with medications or other interventions can make it easier to fall asleep.

Once asleep, pain is masked. This is because the thalamus, a relay nucleus deep within the brain, disconnects the body's sensory input from the cortical surface of the brain from which consciousness arises. The key is to get to sleep: then the experience of pain abates. Moreover, sleep may actually provide pain relief, as is frequently observed with migraine headaches that resolve after rest. To get through the transition, discuss ways to optimize pain relief with your health care provider.

Do not overlook the role of coexisting sleep, psychiatric, and medical disorders that cause pain, especially if you are struggling. By tackling any of these issues, if they are present, you may make lasting improvements that can be very helpful to your long-term health.

Health Impacts and Consequences of Poor Sleep

Sleep not only impacts how someone feels during the day, but poor sleep has long-term consequences affecting health and well-being. Insomnia is a known risk factor for serious impairments in daily function. Moreover, the effects of sleep deprivation may influence health in unexpected and expansive ways.

Now that the shadow of insomnia has begun to be lifted, it is important to celebrate what an important change this is. Persistent, unrelenting insomnia is a significant risk factor for other problems. Beyond the impacts on mood described above, it is linked to the development of other psychiatric disorders including bipolar disorder, attention deficit hyperactivity disorder (ADHD), and schizophrenia. It is linked to higher incidences of alcohol or drug abuse, as afflicted individuals attempt to cope with the disorder. It leads to significant social and occupational dysfunction, affecting the success of relationships and professional pursuits.

Beyond these real-world consequences, the toll of **sleep deprivation** also begins to undermine health. The inability to obtain adequate rest may have profound effects:

- Daytime sleepiness may be noted.
- As mentioned, impairments of the frontal lobe affect mood and executive functions.
- Sleep deprivation leads to poor concentration and short-term memory impairment. This affects work performance and contributes to errors, accidents, and even disasters (such as the crash of the Exxon Valdez, the Chernobyl nuclear meltdown, and frequent transit catastrophes).

- Visual hallucinations affect 80 percent of sleep-deprived people and paranoia may occur in about 2 percent of those with inadequate rest.
- Pain intolerance increases and chronic pain disorders may be noted.
- Changes in growth hormone and thyroid hormone may impact the repair of the body's tissues. Children may not reach their full growth potential.
- Weight gain may occur due to abnormal regulation of appetite hormones, including leptin and ghrelin.
- There is an increased risk of cardiovascular disease, including heart attacks. Those who sleep less than 5 hours have 2 to 3 times the risk of a heart attack.
- The immune system is unable to function normally and the risk of infection (including with the rhinovirus that causes colds) increases and the ability to fight off infections is compromised.
- Most concerning, sleep deprivation that is associated with shift work seems to increase the risk of colorectal and breast cancer.

Though the impairments affect nearly every aspect of health, there is good news: recovery occurs quickly. There is considerable evidence that even one night of improved sleep can reverse the effects of sleep deprivation. It is not possible to undo damage endured from prior sleep loss, but by fixing insomnia and optimizing sleep quality and quantity, it is possible to change direction and head down a path toward better health.

Improving Sleep Hygiene and Habits

Though most people with insomnia have already made significant efforts to optimize their sleep habits, it is necessary to review a little basic advice to ensure that a minor change that may be helpful is not left undone. Sometimes called **sleep hygiene**, these are the basic recommendations that can be found in news articles, self-help books, and on the lips of friends and family the world over.

These particular guidelines are adapted from the National Sleep Foundation. Take a moment to review this list and see if any of these changes may be helpful to you as you tidy up the last few aspects of improving your sleep health:

1. **Maintain a regular sleep-wake schedule.** As reinforced as part of this program, observe a fixed wake time and go to bed feeling sleepy, at about the same time every day. Keep to this schedule, even on weekends.

2. **Don't eat too close to bedtime.** Food prompts the release of insulin, which may make it hard to fall asleep. Heavy meals and spicy foods may also cause heartburn while lying down. It is recommended that 2 hours pass between the last meal and bedtime.

3. **Reserve the bedroom as a space only for sleep.** Do not watch television, use a computer, or keep the phone in the bedroom. Remove all electronics. Do not work in the bed. Avoid prolonged wakefulness in bed. Make the bedroom dark and quiet. Keep the temperature cool to promote sleep.

4. **Exercise regularly, but avoid aerobic exercise at least 3 hours before going to bed.** An increase in body temperature can make it hard to fall asleep. If this is the only time in your

day that is available to exercise, and it is not impacting your sleep, an exception can be made.

5. **Pay attention to the timing of your intake of caffeine, nicotine, and alcohol.** Do not drink caffeine for about 6 hours before going to bed. If you are especially sensitive, consider stopping consumption by noon or even entirely. Alcohol consumption should end in time to allow 1 hour to pass for each alcoholic drink before going to bed. Nicotine is a stimulant that undermines sleep, so consider efforts to quit smoking.

6. **Avoid taking naps.** Sleeping during the day will diminish the ability to sleep at night. Naps can make up for lost sleep time, but may worsen insomnia.

When to Seek Further Help

If this chapter has raised some concerns for you about underlying conditions that may be impacting your ability to sleep normally, it might be time to reach out to a professional for further help. This is especially important if you feel like you are not making sufficient progress toward your goals despite careful adherence to the recommendations of the program.

Consider initially speaking with your health care provider for additional evaluation and treatment. Mood disorders may require assistance from a psychologist or psychiatrist. It may also be helpful to seek a referral to a board-certified sleep medicine physician for additional testing. To find a sleep center accredited by the American Academy of Sleep Medicine near you, go to: sleepeducation.org/find-a-facility.

After a formal consultation, the sleep medicine specialist can arrange appropriate testing, including either a home sleep apnea test or an in-center diagnostic polysomnogram. If sleep apnea is identified based on this testing, treatment with a continuous positive airway pressure (CPAP) machine, an oral appliance from a specialty dentist, weight optimization, or limited surgical options can be considered.

If you are interested in working with an in-person sleep psychologist to optimize your response to cognitive behavioral therapy for insomnia (CBT-I), which is the basis for this program, consider contacting a local sleep center or search for psychologists online who are members of the American Board of Sleep Medicine at: absm.org/BSMSpecialists.aspx.

There is plenty of help out there with credentialed specialists with the training and expertise to provide assistance—so if you are struggling, don't be afraid to reach out.

Further Sleep Extension to Meet Program Goals

It is time again to review your current sleep log and make adjustments to your sleep schedule for the week ahead. Review your initial program goals. What further changes are necessary for you to ultimately meet these goals? Review the strengths and weaknesses from the assessment you did at the beginning of this chapter. Consider what incremental changes are needed this week to make further progress toward those final ends. It is likely that the bedtime needs to be advanced a little earlier this week so that you can get a little more sleep and move closer to meeting your sleep needs. (It may be helpful to review the sleep extension instructions from p. 75, as necessary.)

By reviewing your most recent sleep log, you may note sustained improvements in the average time that it is taking to fall asleep or the total time that you are spending awake at night. Sleepiness may be gradually improving, especially compared to the first week of sleep consolidation, but it may not be resolved, as you likely still need more sleep. To obtain this additional sleep, it is important to continue to move your bedtime earlier incrementally, if your sleep efficiency allows it.

As was done last week, use the instructions previously provided to calculate your current sleep efficiency. If appropriate, continue to adjust either your wake time or bedtime incrementally. If you are waking up at your goal, but need more sleep based on the sleep efficiency calculation, go to bed 15 minutes earlier this week. These adjustments will continue over the next weeks until you have met your sleep needs and are feeling fully rested during the day. As this time is added back, you will notice that you are feeling better rested without a recurrence of insomnia. If the sleep efficiency takes a dip, with more time needed to fall asleep or spent awake in the night, this could be a sign that your time in bed has started to exceed your actual sleep needs. Use the sleep efficiency instructions to make any adjustments that may be needed. Beyond the changes in the timing of your sleep, recommit yourself to the other treatment goals that require a little additional attention or effort this week.

Conclusion

This week we assessed the strengths and weaknesses of your adherence to the treatment recommendations in order to identify areas of improvement as the program enters its final phase. We learned about the causes of fatigue that extend beyond sleep, including the role of diet, exercise, medical conditions, and medications. We explored the relationship between persistent insomnia and underlying disorders that affect sleep—including, importantly, obstructive sleep apnea—as well as the roles of untreated mood problems (like anxiety and depression) and chronic pain. We reviewed the significant impacts on long-term health and well-being in the context of sleep deprivation. We discovered ways to optimize sleep hygiene by identifying additional factors that may compromise sleep. After considering conditions that may contribute to insomnia and undermine response to insomnia therapy, we also identified when to seek further professional help and resources that are available. Finally, we reviewed your current sleep log to continue the process of sleep extension based on sleep efficiency.

Week 5 Goals:

- Continue keeping a sleep log (p. 141) to track your progress.
- Observe a fixed wake time by getting up at the same time every day with an alarm clock. Set the alarm clock for a goal wake time of _____.
- Do not check the clock at night. Set the alarm and turn or cover it at night to avoid clock checking.

- Get 15 to 30 minutes of morning sunlight upon awakening (or at sunrise).
- Avoid taking naps unless required for safety (and keep them brief if needed).
- New goal bedtime at _____ with lights out immediately. Spend 60 minutes relaxing before bedtime (using list for ideas). If necessary, stay up later until feeling sleepy.
- If awake for more than 15 minutes at night, by your estimate, get up and go to another room and do something relaxing until feeling sleepy and then come back to bed.
- Continue to use cognitive therapy, scheduled worry time, and relaxation techniques as needed.
- If you are using sleeping pills, continue to taper or discontinue these medications with the supervision of your prescribing doctor.

Note: After your next week of sleep extension, return to this text and begin the final book chapter.

Lasting Change and Preventing Relapse

Reflection: Most Helpful Elements
Education: Capitalizing on Gains, Preventing Relapses
Goal Setting: Lasting Change

Learning Objectives:

- Reflect on the program's components and identify those that have been most helpful in improving your sleep.
- Review the progress that has been made over the last weeks by revisiting your program goals and identify areas that need additional attention.
- Optimize your sleep schedule and continue to make adjustments as needed to improve sleep efficiency and meet sleep needs.

- Learn how to sustain the gains that have been made and prevent future relapses of chronic insomnia by answering some frequently asked questions.
- Use the guidelines, skills, and information you have learned to sleep normally the rest of your life.

Reflecting on the Most Helpful Aspects of the Program

As we enter the final week of the *Sleep Through Insomnia* program, assuming all has gone according to plan, it may seem hard to believe the transformation in your sleep that has occurred. Over the past weeks, education and changes rooted in science have hopefully given you the skills needed to sleep more normally. The advice at times may have seemed counterintuitive—if you can't sleep, go to bed later—but the results are real. It has taken time, and there may still be more work to do, but you are on the path to resolving insomnia. Now is the time to identify what helped you the most so that you may sustain these gains over the rest of your life.

Take a moment to review and reflect on what aspects of this program have been especially helpful to you. Was there a "Eureka!" moment when something clicked for you? Did you discover a specific change that really made all the difference to your sleep? This is undoubtedly highly personal and will vary based on your individual needs and situation. Consider how these various treatment components may have improved your sleep and highlight those that have been most helpful:

- Learning more about sleep: understanding the sleep drive, circadian rhythm, and causes of insomnia.
- Tracking sleep patterns with a sleep log to identify relationships.
- Considering sleep needs and reducing time in bed to reflect the ability to sleep by calculating sleep efficiency.
- Waking up at the same time every day.
- Getting 15 to 30 minutes of morning sunlight upon awakening
- Going to bed when feeling sleepy.
- Consolidating sleep by reducing the total amount of time in bed.
- Getting out of bed if not feeling sleepy to strengthen conditioning.
- Spending 60 minutes before bedtime relaxing to improve the ability to fall asleep.
- Challenging sleep-related thoughts that may not have a basis in reality.
- Learning about mindfulness, breathing techniques, progressive muscle relaxation, and guided imagery.
- Using relaxation techniques as a means to distract the mind at sleep onset.
- Scheduling worry time daily to productively manage stress and anxiety.
- Accepting that sleep cannot be forced and not trying so hard to make it happen.
- Reserving the bed and bedroom as a space for sleep and sex.
- Eliminating naps during the day.
- Not looking at the clock or checking the time at night.
- Reducing caffeine, alcohol, or nicotine use to improve sleep.

- Understanding the relative ineffectiveness and dangers of using sleeping pills.
- Gradually tapering and stopping the use of sleeping pills.
- Learning about other causes of fatigue.
- Identifying and treating coexisting sleep, mood, and medical disorders.
- Finding pleasurable things to do when unable to sleep.
- Enhancing wakefulness and discovering ways to enjoy mornings.
- Accepting that sleep quality improves even though total sleep time is reduced.
- Feeling hopeful that insomnia will improve and the sleep system can be normalized.

Revisiting Your Program Goals

At the beginning of the program, goals were established to work toward over the weeks that followed. Some of these may have seemed initially far-fetched and all, if met, would indicate a successful completion of the program. Let's take a moment to review these goals from Week 1 and see how you have done.

If you were taking sleeping pills, were you able to taper or discontinue these medications with the help of your prescribing doctor? Are you falling asleep faster at the beginning of the night? Have you had more nights when you fall asleep in less than 20 minutes? Is less time spent awake in the night after awakenings occur? Have you improved your sleep continuity (as measured by sleep efficiency)? Are you getting enough hours of sleep on average to feel rested? Do you still need more sleep to meet your sleep needs? Are you going to bed and getting up when you wanted to? Do you need to continue to adjust your sleep schedule to meet your goals of sleep timing? Have you noticed improvements in your daytime function, especially relating to mood and thinking? Did you discover that you have symptoms suggestive of an underlying sleep disorder? Have you made arrangements to seek further evaluation or to have a sleep study?

No doubt if you have stuck with the program and done your best to adhere to the recommendations, you have made significant improvements. There may still be a little work left to do, and that is not unexpected. This is the ideal time to focus attention on areas that may require additional optimization. Moreover, now is the time to create a sleep schedule to follow until sleep needs are fully met.

Creating a Sleep Schedule to Meet Sleep Needs

It is quite possible that you need to continue to extend your time in bed, as you are not yet meeting your sleep needs. Recall that the average amount of sleep needed by an adult ranges from 7 to 9 hours, and that adults over age 65 years may only need 7 to 8 hours of sleep to feel rested. If you have persistent daytime sleepiness (such as a desire to nap or a tendency to doze when sedentary), or have a sleep efficiency exceeding 85 percent, these adjustments should continue. It may be helpful to create a schedule to follow over the next weeks.

Take this example and adjust it to reflect your goals of bedtime, wake time, and total sleep needs:

Week	Bedtime Goal	Wake Time
1	12:00 a.m.	7:00 a.m.
2	11:45 p.m.	7:00 a.m.
3	11:30 p.m.	7:00 a.m.
4	11:15 p.m.	6:45 a.m.
5	11:00 p.m.	6:30 a.m.
6 and onward	11:00 a.m.	6:30 a.m.

Let's assume that the first week reflects your current sleep schedule. Your sleep efficiency is at 90 percent, and you are having trouble staying awake until midnight. As a result, you choose to continue to advance your bedtime earlier by 15 minutes a week at a time. You keep your wake time fixed and continue to get morning sunlight upon awakening. By week 3, you are feeling completely rested by getting close to 7½ hours of sleep. Your sleep efficiency is stable and insomnia has not recurred. Your day-time sleepiness has resolved and you can stay up to your bedtime easily. You have decided that you would like to get up earlier to go to the gym. Your new goal wake time is 6:30 a.m. Over the next several weeks, you start by setting your alarm 15 minutes earlier (adjust the wake time first). You continue to go to bed when feeling sleepy, and within a few days this bedtime has also moved 15 minutes earlier. The next week you make another adjustment in the wake time by setting the alarm to 6:30 a.m. By the end, you are pleased with your schedule and wish to continue it for the time being.

If at any point you start to make changes to your sleep schedule and your sleep efficiency drops, or insomnia recurs, consider returning to the prior week's schedule. Too much time in bed worsens insomnia. As needed, revisit further sleep consolidation, reducing the time in bed to enhance your ability to sleep. This may also be needed at any point in the future to prevent a relapse of chronic insomnia.

How to Prevent Relapses of Chronic Insomnia

As mentioned previously, you have now learned a set of skills that will help you to sleep better the rest of your life. There may be times that you face a setback. A stressful event in life can make it hard to fall asleep. Fortunately, you can avoid going down the path to chronic insomnia. Simple changes, such as getting up when you can't sleep or going to bed later, may help to reset those bad nights. You have also learned ways to defuse anxious thoughts with scheduled worry time and cognitive therapy and how to employ relaxation techniques to calm the mind at night. It is possible to sustain the gains you have made and prevent future relapses by reviewing the key recommendations that have served you well in this program.

The key is consistency. If at any point you find that you have gotten lax in your observation of these recommendations, start from the top and see where improvement is needed. It may be necessary to become strict in your observation of these rules until things get back on track. When people are sleeping normally, some flexibility is well-tolerated. Rarely, you may even need to repeat sleep consolidation, reducing the time in bed to reflect your current sleep needs (and to as few as 6 hours in bed), and gradually adding the time back week by week.

This is the recipe for good sleep. Take a moment to reflect on these ongoing goals and consider posting this list somewhere to remind you of how to stay on track. If you struggle at any point in the future, come back to it.

Guidelines to Complete Insomnia Therapy

1. Maintain a fixed wake time every day with an alarm and get morning sunlight exposure for 15 to 30 minutes upon awakening.

2. Spend time relaxing for 1 hour prior to bedtime to transition to sleep. Go to bed feeling sleepy with a regular bedtime.

3. If awake for more than 15 minutes in bed, by your estimate, get up and go to another room and do a relaxing activity until feeling sleepy. Then return to the bed to sleep. Reserve the bed for sleep and sex.

4. If persistent difficulty falling, staying, or returning to sleep, delay bedtime to allow only 6 hours of time in bed. As sleep improves, gradually move the bedtime earlier in 15-minute increments one week at a time. Use the sleep efficiency calculation to make these changes if desired.

5. If sleeping well, keep a consistent bedtime and wake time to allow about 7 to 8 hours of rest. Do not take naps.

6. As needed, use relaxation techniques (breathing, progressive muscle relaxation, or guided imagery) and scheduled worry time to calm your mind at night.

Answering a Few Frequently Asked Questions (FAQs)

What if my insomnia recurs?

Recall that you likely have an underlying genetic or neurochemical baseline that may predispose you toward developing difficulty falling or staying asleep. This may be exacerbated by acute triggers and made persistent by untreated sleep or mood disorders. Due to this tendency, be aware that insomnia may indeed recur at some point in the future. Life happens! Do not worry that you have completely lost the gains that you made. You will be able to get yourself back on track by adhering to these very same recommendations. As needed, revisit the program to remind yourself of the skills needed to get back on track.

Do I have to be strict with my schedule forever?

It is unlikely that you have to follow your fixed bedtime and wake time each and every night. Of course, you can always stay up later or get up earlier than your goals. Moreover, some variability is expected in normal sleep. Accept this. Listen to your body. If you are feeling particularly sleepy one night, consider going to bed early. Avoid extending your time in bed too much night after night, however, as this may cause insomnia to recur. As best as you can, try to wake up at the same time every day. If you travel, you may experience jet lag, the same as everyone else, and following specific recommendations for this condition can help reset your sleep more quickly. If you struggle at any point, return to a more strict observation of your schedule.

Can I read in bed?

Many people without insomnia read in bed for 15 to 20 minutes before turning the lights out. This is a comfortable way to transition to sleep. This might also work for you. How do you know? Try it out! If you find that reading is tolerated, keep doing it. If you struggle to get to sleep after turning out the light, it may be a sign that it doesn't work for you. You may have to read elsewhere in the house and come to bed with the intent of immediately turning out the lights. Avoid spending prolonged periods lying awake in bed, and reading if it occurs should be kept short. As much as possible, reserve the bed for sleep and sex and exclude all other activities.

What should I do if I can't get to sleep?

This is one of the key concerns of people with insomnia, especially if there is a component of anxiety. As discussed, the best solution is to engage in a quiet, relaxing activity while waiting for the sleep drive to build. This may involve delaying the bedtime. Don't get upset or frustrated, as these feelings will interfere with your ability to fall asleep. Instead, spend the time relaxing and waiting for sleepiness to come. Do not work; engage in an activity that is calming and unproductive. In the buffet of life: choose oatmeal. If you are in bed, give yourself 15 to 20 minutes to fall asleep by your estimate, and if it is not happening, get up and return to bed later when you are feeling sleepy. If you are faced with fewer hours in bed, the sleep quality will be enhanced through consolidation and you may actually feel better rested with less sleep.

If I am still using sleeping pills, will I ever be able to stop them?

Continue to work with your prescribing provider to reduce the use of sleeping pills if this persists. As noted, there can be both physical and psychological dependence on the medications. You may rely on the medicine to sleep, and feel nervous at the thought of not having the sleep aid. Beyond this, there is normal rebound insomnia that occurs as the dose is reduced or the medication is stopped. Try to observe additional sleep consolidation, reducing the time in bed and going to bed feeling extra sleepy, as you cut the dose. You may take half a tablet as you go to bed, and keep the second half of the tablet on your nightstand. If you need it, it is there, but hopefully you can fall asleep without it. As you work at this, you may find that you need the pills less often and can gradually stop using sleep aids completely.

Why do I need to focus on my wake time?

When insomnia occurs, it is not unusual to focus efforts on falling asleep and protecting the bedtime routine. As you have likely experienced, this is not helpful. Instead, this additional attention makes it even harder to fall asleep. Instead, place your attention on observing a fixed wake time every day, including weekends. Set an alarm to keep this anchored and stable. Don't allow yourself to sleep in if you have a particularly bad night. You will be sleepy during the day, but sleep better the next night. As part of your morning routine, get up immediately upon awakening and get 15 to 30 minutes of morning sunlight as soon as possible (or at sunrise). This helps to strengthen both the natural sleep drive and the circadian rhythm.

Are there long-term consequences to sleeping less?

It may seem like an odd question, but people with insomnia often worry about the long-term effects of reduced sleep time. Would you ask if there were consequences to not eating as much as someone else? You should sleep, and eat, as much as your body needs to function at its best. Some people have lower sleep needs. The concern comes when you are sleeping less than you need to feel rested. If you struggle with daytime sleepiness, power your day with caffeine, fall asleep unintentionally when sedentary, or let life dictate how much you sleep, you are likely to face the effects of sleep deprivation. If you get enough sleep to feel rested, even if it is only 7 hours, you need not worry about these potential harms.

What if I need more help?

If at any point you find that you are struggling, consider reaching out for professional help. As discussed in the last chapter, meeting with your health care provider, a board-certified sleep medicine physician, or a behavioral psychologist may be necessary. This program is based on the latest advances in science and years of clinical experience with hundreds of patients, but sometimes talking to someone about your particular situation may prove necessary. Further testing and treatment may be required to optimize your sleep and response to insomnia therapy.

Conclusion: A Final Word from Dr. Peters

This week we reviewed the major components of the *Sleep Through Insomnia* program and identified those that have been most helpful to improving your sleep. You have reflected on the progress you have made toward your goals and have made plans to continue to adjust your schedule to optimize sleep efficiency and meet your sleep needs. We have learned how to sustain these gains and prevent future relapses to avoid chronic insomnia. We have also answered some of the frequently asked questions that may come up moving forward.

It is my sincere hope that this insomnia program has been helpful to you. You have now learned a set of guidelines and skills that, if consistently employed, may help you to sleep better the rest of your life. Research suggests that the improvement is sustained for years after the conclusion of therapy. Use this information to the benefit of your sleep and health. Make the most of the new life that you have: enjoy time with family and friends, be productive in your profession, and serve your community. Moreover, let others who are suffering from insomnia know about this program so that they may similarly benefit from its use.

 Sleep well, be happy.
Dr. Peters

Ongoing Sleep Goals:

- As needed, continue keeping a sleep log to track your progress.
- Observe a fixed wake time by getting up at the same time every day with an alarm clock. Set the alarm clock for a goal wake time of _____.
- Do not check the clock at night. Set the alarm and turn or cover it at night to avoid clock checking.
- Get 15 to 30 minutes of morning sunlight upon awakening (or at sunrise).
- Avoid taking naps unless required for safety (and keep them brief if needed).
- New goal bedtime at _____ with lights out immediately. Spend 60 minutes relaxing before bedtime (using list for ideas). If necessary, stay up later until feeling sleepy.
- If awake for more than 15 minutes at night, by your estimate, get up and go to another room and do something relaxing until feeling sleepy and then come back to bed.
- Continue to use cognitive therapy, scheduled worry time, and relaxation techniques as needed.
- If you are using sleeping pills, continue to taper or discontinue these medications with the supervision of your prescribing doctor.

Sleep Logs

For access to a free set of downloadable and printable sleep logs, visit BrandonPetersMD.com/sleeplogs.

Otherwise, consider following the format on the next page, recording 7 days of information on each week's sleep log.

CBT-I Week #_____	Today's Date: _____ /_____ /_____
1. List any sleep aids you took (medication name, dose, time taken).	
2. What time did you get into bed?	___:___ p.m./a.m.
3. What time did you turn out the lights and try to go to sleep?	___:___ p.m./a.m.
4. How long did it take to fall asleep?	_____ min(s)
5. How many times did you wake?	_____ time(s)
6. In total, how long spent awake?	_____ min(s)
7. What time did you finally awaken?	___:___ a.m.
8. What time did you get out of bed?	___:___ a.m.
9. In total, how long did you sleep?	_____ hour(s)
10. What was the quality of your sleep (1=very poor … 5=very good)?	
11. How long did you nap yesterday?	_____ min(s)
12. Comments (if applicable):	

CBT-I Week #_____	Today's Date: ____ / ____ / _____
1. List any sleep aids you took (medication name, dose, time taken).	
2. What time did you get into bed?	___:___ p.m./a.m.
3. What time did you turn out the lights and try to go to sleep?	___:___ p.m./a.m.
4. How long did it take to fall asleep?	_____ min(s)
5. How many times did you wake?	_____ time(s)
6. In total, how long spent awake?	_____ min(s)
7. What time did you finally awaken?	___:___ a.m.
8. What time did you get out of bed?	___:___ a.m.
9. In total, how long did you sleep?	_____ hour(s)
10. What was the quality of your sleep (1=very poor ... 5=very good)?	
11. How long did you nap yesterday?	_____ min(s)
12. Comments (if applicable):	

CBT-I Week #_____ Today's Date: ____ / ____ / _____	
1. List any sleep aids you took (medication name, dose, time taken).	
2. What time did you get into bed?	___:___ p.m./a.m.
3. What time did you turn out the lights and try to go to sleep?	___:___ p.m./a.m.
4. How long did it take to fall asleep?	_____ min(s)
5. How many times did you wake?	_____ time(s)
6. In total, how long spent awake?	_____ min(s)
7. What time did you finally awaken?	___:___ a.m.
8. What time did you get out of bed?	___:___ a.m.
9. In total, how long did you sleep?	_____ hour(s)
10. What was the quality of your sleep (1=very poor ... 5=very good)?	
11. How long did you nap yesterday?	_____ min(s)
12. Comments (if applicable):	

CBT-I Week #_____	**Today's Date:** ____ / ____ / _____
1. List any sleep aids you took (medication name, dose, time taken).	
2. What time did you get into bed?	___:___ p.m./a.m.
3. What time did you turn out the lights and try to go to sleep?	___:___ p.m./a.m.
4. How long did it take to fall asleep?	_____ min(s)
5. How many times did you wake?	_____ time(s)
6. In total, how long spent awake?	_____ min(s)
7. What time did you finally awaken?	___:___ a.m.
8. What time did you get out of bed?	___:___ a.m.
9. In total, how long did you sleep?	_____ hour(s)
10. What was the quality of your sleep (1=very poor … 5=very good)?	
11. How long did you nap yesterday?	_____ min(s)
12. Comments (if applicable):	

CBT-I Week #_____ Today's Date: ____ / ____ / _____	
1. List any sleep aids you took (medication name, dose, time taken).	
2. What time did you get into bed?	___:___ p.m./a.m.
3. What time did you turn out the lights and try to go to sleep?	___:___ p.m./a.m.
4. How long did it take to fall asleep?	_____ min(s)
5. How many times did you wake?	_____ time(s)
6. In total, how long spent awake?	_____ min(s)
7. What time did you finally awaken?	___:___ a.m.
8. What time did you get out of bed?	___:___ a.m.
9. In total, how long did you sleep?	_____ hour(s)
10. What was the quality of your sleep (1=very poor ... 5=very good)?	
11. How long did you nap yesterday?	_____ min(s)
12. Comments (if applicable):	

CBT-I Week #_____	Today's Date: ____ / ____ / ____
1. List any sleep aids you took (medication name, dose, time taken).	
2. What time did you get into bed?	___:___ p.m./a.m.
3. What time did you turn out the lights and try to go to sleep?	___:___ p.m./a.m.
4. How long did it take to fall asleep?	_____ min(s)
5. How many times did you wake?	_____ time(s)
6. In total, how long spent awake?	_____ min(s)
7. What time did you finally awaken?	___:___ a.m.
8. What time did you get out of bed?	___:___ a.m.
9. In total, how long did you sleep?	_____ hour(s)
10. What was the quality of your sleep (1=very poor ... 5=very good)?	
11. How long did you nap yesterday?	_____ min(s)
12. Comments (if applicable):	

References

Belleville G. "Mortality hazard associated with anxiolytic and hypnotic use in the National Population Health Survey." *Can J Psychiatry* 2010;55:558-567.

Borbély AA. "A two process model of sleep regulation." *Hum Neurobiol* 1982;1:195-204.

Chong Y *et al.* "Prescription sleep aid use among adults: United States, 2005-2010." *National Center for Health Statistics data brief.* August 2013;127.

Durmer JS *et al.* "Pediatric Sleep Medicine." *Continuum Neurol* 2007; 13(3):153-200.

Glass J *et al.* "Sedative hypnotics in older people with insomnia: meta-analysis of risks and benefits." *BMJ* 2005;331:1169.

Guilleminault C, Eldridge FL, and Dement WC. "Insomnia with sleep apnea: a new syndrome." *Science* 1973 Aug 31;181(4102)856-8.

Hausken AM *et al.* "Use of anxiolytic or hypnotic drugs and total mortality in a general middle-aged population." *Pharmacoepidemiol Drug Saf* 2007;16:913-918.

Iliff JJ *et al.* "Brain-wide pathway for waste clearance captured by contrast-enhanced MRI." *J Clin Invest* 2013 Mar;123(3):1299–1309.

International Classification of Sleep Disorders. American Academy of Sleep Medicine. 3rd edition. 2014.

Kessler RC *et al.* "Insomnia and the performance of US workers: results from the America insomnia survey." *Sleep* 2011;34116171.

Kripke DF *et al.* "Hypnotics' association with mortality or cancer: a matched cohort study." *BMJ Open* 2012;2:e000850.

Mallon L *et al.* "Is usage of hypnotics associated with mortality?" *Sleep Med* 2009;10:279–286.

Ohayon M, Carskadon MA, Guilleminault C, *et al.* "Meta-analysis of quantitative sleep parameters from childhood to old age in healthy individuals: developing normative sleep values across the human lifespan." *Sleep* 2004;27:1255–1273.

Peters BR. "Ethical considerations in sleep medicine." *FOCUS: The Journal of Lifelong Learning.* American Psychiatric Association. 2014;Volume XII(1):64–67.

Peters BR. "Irregular bedtimes and awakenings." *Sleep Medicine Clinics,* Elsevier. 2014;9(4):481–489.

Peters BR. "Trained sleep physicians can effectively administer cognitive behavioral therapy for insomnia (CBT-I) in the clinical setting." *SLEEP* 2015, Seattle, WA, June 2015.

Peters BR. "High incidence of obstructive sleep apnea noted in an older population presenting for cognitive behavioral therapy for insomnia (CBT-I) treatment." *SLEEP* 2015, Seattle, WA, June 2015.

Peters BR. "Untreated sleep apnea masked by sleeping pills undermines efficacy of insomnia therapy." *SLEEP* 2017, Boston, MA, June 2017.

Peters BR and Kushida CA. "Normal sleep." In: Avidan A, ed., *Review of Sleep Medicine,* 4th edition. Philadelphia: Elsevier. 2017;773–788.

Peters BR, Sha SJ, and Yaffe K. "Sleep and cognitive impairment." In: Miglis MG, ed., *Sleep and Neurologic Disease*. San Diego: Academic Press. 2017;73–88.

Pigeon WR *et al*. "Meta-analysis of sleep disturbance and suicidal thoughts and behaviors." *J Clin Psychiatry* 2012;73:e1160-e1167.

Qaseem A *et al*. "Management of chronic insomnia disorder in adults: a clinical practice guideline from the American College of Physicians." *Ann Intern Med* 2016;165(2):125-133.

Sateia MJ *et al*. "Clinical practice guideline for the pharmacologic treatment of chronic insomnia in adults: an American Academy of Sleep Medicine clinical practice guideline." *J Clin Sleep Med* 2017;13(2):307-349.

Schutte-Rodin S *et al*. "Clinical guidelines for the evaluation and management of chronic insomnia in adults." *J Clin Sleep Med* 2008;4(5):487-504.

Siebern AT and Manber R. "New developments in cognitive behavioral therapy as the first-line treatment of insomnia." *Psychol Res Behav Manag* 2011;4:21-28.

Spielman AJ, Caruso, L, and Glovinsky PG. "A behavioral perspective on insomnia." *Psychiatr Clin North Am* 1987;10:541-553.

Taylor DJ *et al*. "Insomnia as a health risk factor." *Behav Sleep Med* 2003;1:227-247.

Wade AG. "The societal costs of insomnia." *Neuropsychiatr Dis Treat*. 2011:7:1-18.

About the Author

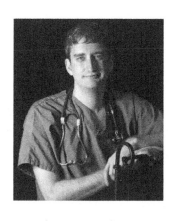 Brandon R. Peters, MD, is a board-certified neurologist and sleep medicine specialist who currently practices at Virginia Mason Medical Center in Seattle. He is also a clinical faculty affiliate at Stanford University's School of Medicine in the Department of Psychiatry and Behavioral Sciences. He previously practiced in Novato, California, at Pulmonary and Sleep Associates of Marin. He has worked in sleep medicine since college, with extensive clinical and research experiences in the field.

Dr. Peters worked in clinical sleep medicine and was trained as a polysomnographic technician prior to starting medical school. His published research includes study of the sleep habits of university students, circadian rhythm disorders in the blind, abnormal sleep behaviors called parasomnias, and sleep ethics.

He was an award-winning journalist in college. His extensive sleep-related writing over the past decade includes more than 1,000 articles on Verywell.com, book chapters, and countless other contributions. He lectures internationally on sleep, frequently appears on radio programs and in other media, and works as a business consultant for related industries.

Dr. Peters received a bachelor of arts degree in biology and English from Seattle Pacific University in Seattle. He also studied medieval and Renaissance literature at Oxford University in England. As noted, Dr. Peters received polysomnographic training to become a sleep technologist at the Swedish Sleep Medicine Institute in Seattle. He went on to receive his medical degree from Oregon Health & Science University in Portland. He completed his neurology residency at the University of Minnesota in Minneapolis. He did his sleep medicine fellowship at Stanford University in Palo Alto, California, viewed internationally as the world's leading training program for sleep disorders medicine. He was additionally trained at Stanford as a practitioner of cognitive behavioral therapy for insomnia (CBT-I).

For more information, please visit BrandonPetersMD.com.

Made in the USA
Las Vegas, NV
26 December 2022

64115830R00098